Cover and interior designs were curated using Canva Pro.

Back cover photo credit to Angela Divine Photography.

ISBN (eBook): 978-1-998393-15-2
ISBN (Paperback): 978-1-998393-16-9
ISBN (Hardcover): 978-1-998393-17-6

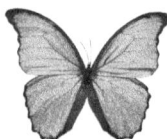

**A.I. Free.
Made with love by a Human.**

Contents

This book is dedicated to Carson and Elle. Thank you for helping me see the beauty in evolving. You have shaped me into the mom and woman I am today.

Stand in your light
and beauty.

♡ Casie

INTRODUCTION

D id you know that being born into this world means that you are perfect as you are? I didn't know that to be true. But the truth is that you—and I—were created and came here because of something greater. Call it God, call it Universe, call it Source, call it whatever you want, but it was more than just a serendipitous, random act that brought you here. In your perfection, you are suited and created for your unique purpose to be fulfilled in this life.

Yet, how is it that you could move from a place of true perfection as a young, carefree girl to feeling like you are, on some level, not enough? This not-enough-ness certainly doesn't come to the forefront day in and day out, but you feel it. You may call it "imposter syndrome" or "self criticism." Maybe you've felt not pretty enough, not thin enough, not successful enough, not stylish enough. Perhaps you think that you aren't driving a nice enough car or that you do not have enough income. Maybe you haven't done enough in the eyes of your boss, and that's why you were passed up for promotion. However it manifests in your life, the not-enough-ness you feel is normal, given the huge gap between where you once were and where you are living today.

The good news is that it doesn't have to be this way. Not anymore. Starting today, you get to move from a place of not feeling beautiful enough—particularly as you age and your body changes—into your unique Age of Beauty.

Through these pages, we will bridge the gap by understanding where you are relative to where you once were, and where you desire to get back to in order to feel whole, complete, beautiful, and confident. Perhaps again, perhaps for the first time ever. I will then offer understandable, relatable, and practical steps to help you move from where you are to where you want to be, so you can truly, deeply feel and believe that you are in your Age of Beauty, regardless of what is happening in your life, your age, or the challenges you face. This is a journey that I, too, have walked.

This book differs in that it is not going to offer you the latest beauty and wellness trends to help you feel more confident as you age. Plenty of that is already available to you. Instead, this will be a shift, a "letting go" of the need to buy, have, or do the latest thing in order to feel beautiful enough. Instead, you are invited to journey inward to remember who you are as a woman. Doing this will require some unlearning of beliefs about yourself that you've acquired along the way. It is a deep, yet necessary, dive into closing the gap between your true value and what you often feel. It is the path toward feeling your best, despite what is happening in your external world.

If you're worried that I'm going to ask you to put down your favorite anti-aging cream or cancel your next Botox appointment, don't be. Rest assured that this is a "both, and" book; you will finally feel fully beautiful—inside and out. If that includes continuing with all the latest and greatest, so be it. You get to be both deeply certain of your internal beauty, *and* maximize your outward beauty.

Through this easy-to-understand, see-yourself-in-my-shoes perspective, I will become your trusted expert in learning how to Age with Beauty. More specifically, you will learn how to Age with Grace, Fire, Wisdom, and Self-Love. So, if you're ready to finally feel like the beautiful woman you are, and live into your confident badassery, then buckle up! It's going to be a great ride, and baby, you're worth it!

Be sure to have your companion *Age of Beauty* workbook by your side as you read through each chapter. To maximize your learning and benefit from this book, I recommend reading one chapter per week. First, read a chapter, then utilize the companion workbook. Each week will offer ways to reflect on and reframe beliefs that no longer serve you, and allow time to process how you want to be living and loving yourself, now and as you age.

Before diving into Chapter 1, go to your workbook and complete the Introduction section. This will help you to become clear on where you are, and to set your intention for this journey.

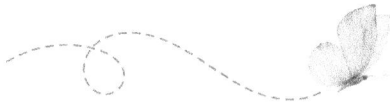

PART ONE

THE CONDITIONING

Chapter One

The Tapestry

From the moment you were born, you were perfect. The moment you were placed in your mother's arms, your father's embrace, your doctor's sturdy hands, a never-before-felt level of love filled your parents' hearts as they gazed at you. You brought newfound joy to your parents, to random patrons in the check-out line at the grocery store, and to the world. When they laid eyes on you, they knew with every cell in their being that this love and connection was miraculous and right. All they knew, and all you knew, was love: pure and perfect love.

Even if you were not fortunate enough to be born to loving parents, their limited capacity does not detract from the truth that you were born exactly as you were meant to be, for a purpose that only you can serve. Their limitations were about them. They were never about you. You were perfectly created, at the ideal time, for a purpose only you can fulfill in your time here on Earth. There is no one else like you—truly, purely, uniquely you—and that knowing makes you perfect.

And then something changed.

What changed is the tapestry you were born into—the societal norms and expectations that have shaped and formed you. There is nothing wrong with these norms, but we have to understand them to get context for what started to shift and why.

The very first inkling was, perhaps, when you cried and your needs were not met right away. Not because your parents didn't care, but because they didn't fully understand if your cries meant you were tired, hungry, hurting, or sitting in a soaked diaper. Perhaps you recall a time when your mother, who was exhausted and going through her own hormonal imbalances, snapped at you or couldn't get to you quickly enough. Maybe your stressed-out dad didn't have time to hear your stories between his business calls.

These early experiences began a shift from love to fear.

One of my first inklings was from when I was around three-years-old and had been picking my nose for quite some time. I must have learned that this was unacceptable behavior from the critical eye of my mom, or the horrified looks from the people in the grocery store line who used to look at me with loving smiles. When I saw it drew disappointed, disgusted faces from those I loved and depended on, I learned how to deal with the behavior. I learned that if I at least hid behind the couch and wiped it down low, I could still be who I was (the clean girl with the freshly-picked nose) *and* be fully loved by others. That lasted until I picked and wiped in what I thought was my usual spot in the living room, but this time a bit too high, and my mom, who kept a meticulously clean home, discovered the crusted evidence. I thought quickly, and blamed it on my one-year-old brother who was barely toddling around. Luckily, she bought it and I was off the hook. This is the first time I can remember hiding, even lying, about who I was for the sake of fitting in, for the sake of receiving "unconditional" love.

Take a moment to think back to your first experience of not being loved and accepted for the full (maybe nose-picking and all) girl that you were. Now, I invite you to think of other times in your life where you received this message in other ways. Perhaps it came in the form of a comment from a parent about your weight, or a thoughtless, "We don't eat that." Maybe a "cool kid" in seventh grade laughed at your outfit from the bleachers and whispered to another popular girl. Or did you see raised eyebrows in a meeting after you offered your "not-so-well-thought-out" input? The truth is, over your lifetime you've had millions of pieces of feedback that have slowly moved you further away from the joy, unconditional love, child-like freedom, and "completeness" that you felt; they have moved you from the beauty of who you truly were into a place of lack. From love to fear. Then layer onto the feedback from the beauty industry and, man, it gets messy!

"Maybe she's born with it. Maybe it's Maybelline," was a message etched into my early subconscious. Since I was clearly not the flawless, matte-skinned supermodel in *Seventeen* magazine, I didn't think I was "born with it," and therefore needed that bright pink blush and thick concealer for my acne. In this fear-based selling model of not-enough-ness, you too were told, and subsequently accepted, that you weren't one of the lucky ones who was "born with it." So, you needed it too, to "make up" for what you lacked. You were incomplete without the beauty industry's help.

You see, fear is what taps into your primal need to feel love and acceptance. Since that gap was created early on and seemed to widen, of course you needed to spend your money on Maybelline makeup, Aquanet, and Guess jeans. These products made you feel as though whatever was missing inside you could be filled.

Fear sells, and fear is what makes beauty and wellness companies billions of dollars, year after year. Fear makes you believe you need that lip gloss, cellulite cream, fuller-coverage makeup, and bronzing powder in order to somehow be appealing—and accepted. You begin to believe you need these things, that are outside yourself, to bridge the gap between your place of less-than and limited worth to become the woman who is complete.

But you are smart, so you quickly adapted. You learned that you could control some of this, so you adjusted course and started to buy what you needed to feel beautiful and whole. Maybe you started to hide certain parts of yourself, ensured straight-As despite the difficulty of school, or remained quiet in the meeting unless you knew, without a doubt, that what you were about to share was both safe and right. For a moment, those little things helped. And that helpful moment isn't bad at all. We feel temporarily beautiful or confident. The problem, however, is that it is a quick hit that doesn't last. With the barrage of messages showing us the next thing we need, or how we need to act differently in order to be accepted, the moment quickly fades.

For me, to be a girl and be "beautiful" meant being quiet, smiling, and looking pretty. It meant I had to work hard, and focus on others' needs ahead of my own. It meant I needed to be thin, well-dressed, well-manicured, and well-groomed. It meant putting on makeup everyday and blow drying my unruly pubescent hair straight, just so I could curl it again, but in a more-controlled manner. I got great grades, worked my ass off, and could have passed for a "perfect young adult."

I was loved and accepted for all of this, but I wasn't being myself. Instead, I was focused on what I thought others—and society—wanted and needed of me to check all the boxes and fit the mold. I did all of this to look put together and "beautiful" to the outside world, but I sure as hell didn't feel it on the inside. I felt ashamed. Despite my efforts to perfect all these things, I still felt inadequate. I wasn't being fully me. I was acting to be accepted.

You see, when we begin to shift away from the fullness and truth of who we are, we start to place ourselves in a box of others' expectations and needs that don't fully align with our own. Every time we sense disapproval, we move inward, as if it's our fault, as if the walls of the box are closing in, and our shoulder tension rises.

This process of feeling like the walls were closing in continued, and with it, so did my anxiety. Looking back, I can see that I was frustrated with my parents for their inability to love me as fully as I deserved. I was angry with society too, yet felt helpless to do much about it. I eventually realized that I, like you and everyone else, was doing the very best I could with what I knew. This was both a recognition of how things are and an acceptance that when I love, accept, and forgive others, I have the space to enjoy the same for myself. It starts from within. More on this later.

You, too, have been operating under this landscape, and it's no wonder you feel you are not enough, like you are an imposter who has to hustle for your worth. It's no surprise you feel that your ability to be loved and appreciated is somehow tied to how clean your home is, the title you hold, and how many people show up to your party. Your worth seems tied to how many "likes" you have from your social media post, or how "successful" you are, as defined by the outside world. The problem with this is that it leaves you in a place of constant striving. You are driven to be something more and different than who you truly are. No wonder you are feeling burnt out and tired.

Now layer this in with aging. Ironically, when you were younger and had it "all together," what some might say was the "best it was going to be", you certainly didn't feel that. As you age, this idea of happiness, completeness, and wholeness seems to become fleeting and further away because, inevitably, you develop wrinkles, get gray hair, your metabolism slows, your body changes, and you don't believe you have the same sex appeal you once did.

By all standards in America and the Western World, your worth diminishes as you age.

So, where does this leave you? It leaves many of the women I work with feeling that, even though their lives are great and they've done all the "right" things, they are somehow "not enough." They are confused about how to solve this and what to do next.

At this stage, you may be gaining a bit of clarity, and also a sense of complete overwhelm. You may be thinking, "Oh great, Casie just pointed out all the shit that's wrong with me, society, my parents, and the world. Now what?"

You're right, I have pointed out all the problems that, on some level, you already knew were there, but now you have the chance — and choice — to do something about it.

The question is:

What the hell are you going to do?

You can't change the way you were brought up, your age, the beauty industry, or society. But you can begin to change you. As we move into Part II, we will walk through the steps I've gone through during my life, and now take my clients through to first recognize, then own, their self-worth and beauty.

You have the choice to create a better reality for yourself. Regardless of your age or the changing tides of time, this is your moment to step into your Age of Beauty.

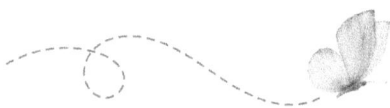

PART TWO

THE CLIMB

Chapter Two

The Striving

You are smart, and were doing the very best you could to operate in a world that didn't see you for the fullness of who you were, so you adapted. You quickly learned that when you were met with discerning eyes or a judgmental comment, you needed to change—that somehow you were the problem. You learned that if you work hard enough, if you hustle enough, if you keep fit enough, you look pretty enough, your hair is long enough, your skin is clear enough, that there's more social love and acceptance. Instead of the discerning, judgmental eye, you received a smile, and captured the gaze of someone, even if it was a creepy old guy. And even though it felt gross, there was part of you that felt accepted and acknowledged.

So, you entered the phase of "striving."

Striving is the part of your life where you move into accomplishing, collecting, and achieving with the promise that if you do it all and do it well, you will be happy. You will get to a place where you feel "enough." This becomes your standard mode of operation.

You work your butt off, and you hit the gym. You try to eat well. You check every single box that tells you that you *should* be happy. You get the husband, the house, the children, and the clothes. Eventually, you get the Botox and keep up with your skin care regimen. You hustle because you know what to do, and you know the gold that is waiting at the end of the rainbow for you: when you get there, you will feel whole and complete. You will feel better.

How do I know all this? How is it that I am recounting your exact experience? Because you and I are the same.

In an article published in *Oprah Daily*, Oprah explains, "...your life whispers to you all the time, if you're paying attention, from the moment you open your eyes in the morning until the moment you go to bed at night... [H]earing those whispers is one of the most integral pieces... of your best life." (Oprah 2021). Yet, we become so busy that we don't have a chance to quiet down enough to hear the whispers that indicate something might be off. That this relentless effort and striving isn't as healthy as we think it might be. It's not good for us because it's not sustainable. You may start to wonder, like I did, if the pot at the end of the rainbow even exists?

Let's face it—we are so busy in this striving phase that all we can do is keep our heads down. We keep going. We keep searching for that approval from our boss, that praise, that promotion, that glimmer of a smile, that acceptance. We don't have a chance to stop or to slow down to listen to these whispers within us.

For me, the whispers came in the form of not being truly happy with what I was doing, and feeling exhausted. I was pumping breastmilk for my son in the car on the way to and from work, feeling that if I was late or skipped a "pumping session," I was falling short. Frantic, I put the milk into the bottle and brought my carry-along freezer with me so that the milk would stay good until I could get it into the refrigerator at the office. Go, go, go. Do, do, do.

The whispers were saying, "You're tired." But it only felt like I was a *bit* out of alignment, and that this was "normal"—to be expected for a woman who was "doing it all." Shouldn't I have been a bit tired and drained with the responsibility of young kids, a full-time job, a marriage, and a waning social life?

Despite how it might feel at times, there is nothing wrong with the striving phase. We all go through it. It's part of what we are taught is going to help us, to serve us well. The only problem is that it isn't all there is.

In our relentless striving, we give our power away. Unknowingly, we give the ultimate say to everyone else in our lives instead of ourselves. We are driven by fear instead of trusting in our inherent worth and ability to be loved. We are subconsciously slipping further from the truth of who we are—our authentic selves.

That is why so many women get to a stage in midlife, after we've done all these things, where we finally look up and ask ourselves, "Why am I still not feeling whole, complete, loved, accepted, and seen as my full self? Something is still off. Something is still not right."

So, what do you do? You shop. You exercise more. You work harder. You may have that extra glass of wine when socializing with friends. You wonder what more you can be doing to keep up. When you get really run down, you cry. Tears seem to bubble up from nowhere when someone looks you in the eye and asks, "How are you *really* doing?" You feel isolated and alone, like you somehow got yourself in this place, like it's your fault. You may start that diet to feel better in your clothes, or stay up late to get back to your colleague. You might keep pumping, and commuting, and cleaning, and organizing, because you believe on some level that you are the problem. If you could just get your life in better order, better control the chaos around you, then—and only then—things would be okay.

My perfectionism was born from noticing and addressing others' needs and expectations ahead of my own, completing tasks early, having given 110%. It was born in my always-put-together style, and in my high-pitched response of, "I'm great, how are you?" If I could keep everyone around me happy, then I'd be happy too, right? I operated under this equation for many years, and it worked reasonably well—until it didn't.

The core problem is that in this state of continuously changing myself to fit the needs of others, my true Self was lost. I spent so much effort and time "controlling" myself and my external environment that I wasn't sure who I really was outside of the labels of: mom, medical device rep, wife, daughter, and friend. It looked like I was good at *being* all of those roles, but in reality, I was *doing* all of those things to keep other people happy, instead of being myself. I was a *human doing*, not a *human being*.

Perhaps you were more of the rebellious type. Maybe you didn't conform like I did but bucked the system. When your dad told you to not leave the house with that crop top on, you tossed it in your backpack anyway and changed in the car. You fought for your voice, to be seen as you truly were. And yet, when you didn't fit the mold (i.e., the expectations of others), you were quickly labeled: She's struggling; She's rebellious; We are worried about her; She's unladylike; Might she be on drugs? or, Is she okay?

Regardless of which path you chose, you decided to comply with or resist a system that wasn't fully seeing you. As a result, resentment, frustration, and anger built. You may have started to point the finger at your husband, boss, or your colleagues for not pulling their weight. Maybe your kids took the brunt of your feelings because you felt like they were being a pain in the ass for not getting out the door in time.

I blamed a lot of people and jobs in my life that caused me a shit-ton of trouble and difficulty at the time. It was easier to blame my resistant, angry feelings on something outside myself instead of looking inward and feeling them. At that point, I don't think I even recognized they were there; it was easier to just blame others. I identified my job, my boss, and my husband as the problems. Again, all of it existed outside me.

I gave all my power away.

What I didn't realize was that I was a contributor. I was creating these feelings for myself by the choices I was making. It was a binary reaction—either comply or resist. Either way, the power rested with everyone but me. I was giving my power away because I didn't recognize my power within, or that I could choose another path outside of "fit in or be rejected." When I was young, the world seemed black and white, as if to be okay, I had to choose one path or the other. I defaulted to the best for me, and you defaulted to the best for you. The love and acceptance we so desperately craved, and also needed for our very survival, was dependent on choosing the "right" path—the one we defaulted to and stuck to. We committed ourselves to either living in or kicking against the box of ever-narrowing walls of expectation.

The confusing thing about striving is that when you did strive, either at work or on the way you looked, you received validation. When you bought that lip gloss, someone said, "Oh my gosh, I love that. Where did you get that?" Maybe the antibiotics you were prescribed to clear your acne finally resulted in someone saying, "Your skin looks great." It didn't matter that your stomach was killing you, or that you ended up switching to Accutane, despite having to sign your life away on waivers of possibly birthing alien kids or ruining your liver. Maybe you got highlights in your hair and someone told you that you look good today, yet you noticed your ends starting to split. Or you bought that great pair of shoes and were rockin' it with that outfit, then heard a validating, "Ooh, I love your look!"—even though you spent more than you felt comfortable with to buy them.

I want to be clear, there was nothing wrong with the way things were. It was a sign of the times and our upbringing. The problem became that we tied our self-worth to it too much. This book is not about negating or avoiding the things that truly help you to feel better, inside and out; the things required for happiness. Social acceptance is a piece of that as it is a part of our culture.

Instead, this book will take you a level deeper, to feel more authentic in who you are, regardless of whether you do those fun, beautifying things, or not. As we move forward, you will be shown a deeper, more satisfying way to enjoy all those aspects of life *and* feel complete. You will feel like you can finally step off of the treadmill of constantly needing to be more, do more, accomplish more, to feel whole. You can feel whole in and of yourself, in a place where all those other things become icing on the cake.

Why?

Because you are complete.

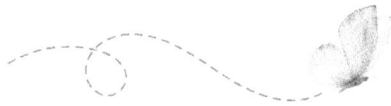

Chapter Three

The Resistance

In this act of striving, climbing, and attempting to do all the things in your life you were told would help you feel beautiful, happy, and enough, you started to feel the disconnect between what you wanted for your life and what was actually happening. This created resistance within you. It created frustration and confusion because life wasn't unfolding in the way it was promised. Doing all of these things "just so" wasn't creating the life you thought it would. Resistance was the result of the disconnect and widening gap between who you really were at your core and the way you were being. When we are out of alignment within ourselves, resistance increases.

In this place of confusion and resistance, you may have started to compare yourself to others. Criticizing or judging them when they had the confidence to speak up in the meeting and you didn't: "Wow, isn't she overly confident. Who does she think she is?"

Perhaps you chose to continue working despite longing to stay home with your children, yet when you met another woman doing so, you quietly questioned if her kids were getting enough interaction with others, and what she did all day. You may have longed to make as much as the woman at work who splurged on designer clothes, yet simultaneously questioned her values and financial responsibility.

This level of comparison and criticism exists because we were brought up in a black and white world. Either you acted right or wrong, good or bad. You were accepted or not. You were doing the right thing, or not, and if someone else veered off course, you judged. If you couldn't keep up, you self-criticized.

In that black and white framework, we started to become part of the tapestry, and part of the challenge. With that came even more resistance because our deeper, authentic selves were crying out to break free from it all. Find another way. Enjoy life more. We didn't feel aligned. Surely there had to be more to break through. Yet within the box of societal norm and expectation, we felt that it was not okay to outwardly express the big feelings inside us. When asked how we were, we responded with, "I'm fine. How are you?" instead of the honest truth.

We dove deeper into work, making sure to reply to emails within an hour or two, so we always seemed on top of it. Maybe we drank a little more than we wanted to. Or shopped to get that outfit that, subconsciously, would help us feel better. We became busy. We became "supermoms." We became the women who could do it all because if we doubled down on striving, which still felt like the only path forward, then we would be enough.

When we weren't quite cutting it—when we came up short, instead of allowing ourselves to feel the true feelings of lack and struggle—we judged ourselves instead: "I must need to work harder," or, "Oh, that was such a stupid question to ask in the meeting." Or we judged others who were acting in a way we would never consider: "I can't believe she would say such a thing," or, "What is she wearing?" It became a mixture of self-judgment and judgment of others for the sake of what felt like survival. Win or lose in this black and white world.

Take a moment and ask yourself which judgment patterns you fall into? And what coping mechanisms do you double down on?

There is no shame in this. You know the things you do habitually, without question. Maybe it's exercising religiously, or weighing yourself daily with the accompanying self-criticism. Whatever your pattern, it was a result of believing that your big feelings outside of this black and white world weren't okay to express. By continuing to focus on the external things you could control to get you closer to "okay" and "enough," you maintained that outward focus on complying with the needs and expectations of the external world. Eventually, those expectations have to increase in order to bridge the gap within yourself. This helped you deal with the fact that you didn't have to face your big, internal feelings. And that made you feel okay. You felt mostly fine.

I'm sure there were days when you felt beautiful—after you got the new handbag or were about to be promoted. But there was probably still an underlying, unrecognized sense of not enough-ness: not beautiful enough, not whole enough, not complete enough. This was all part of a cover to gloss over the underlying shame. In her book, *The Gifts of Imperfection,* Brené Brown explains, "Shame is the most powerful, master emotion. It's the fear that we're not good enough" (Brown 2010). It hits us at the core of who we are as women and as people. It can feel too scary to display any feelings of vulnerability, shame, or lack in a world known to criticize or judge people as being "less than," so instead, we armor up. We strive to achieve or be "perfect" as a way to prevent anyone from seeing our feelings of lack, our underlying shame. We control our external world to the best of our abilities. We strive. And we do it carrying a heavy load of armor along the way. The problem, as Brené identifies in *Daring Greatly,* is, "Wearing armor is a way to protect ourselves from pain, but it also prevents us from experiencing love and joy" (Brown 2012).

Unaware of the growing shame and "not-enoughness" we felt, we worked harder to cover it up. We continued doing as we "should," following the equation we learned, and we developed tension in our shoulders and necks. We became quieter and more calculated about when and how to speak up, analyzing our environment to see if it was truly a safe place to be, and to share. The problem with this is that we are driven by fear-based resistance instead of sharing our true voice, our authentic Self.

For me, this resistance came in the form of judgment and comparison. I would look at myself in the mirror and notice if my hair wasn't as clean, shiny, and smooth as I thought it should be, which created a mild feeling of not being polished enough. I noticed that if my outfit was outdated, or the house cluttered, I didn't feel as confident. An internal voice of judgment seemed to surface as a part of the need for protection, which became my form of perfection. If I fit the mold, did all the things, and seemed as "perfect" as I could be, I would be protected from the judgment of others. I would be safe and happy. Over time, this internal voice became increasingly harsh and critical as it formed part of my safety mechanism. Somehow, I believed that if I was hard enough on myself, I'd do enough and be enough to prevent anyone else from hurting, criticizing, or judging me. That was my armor.

My armor also included constantly comparing myself to other women: "Oh, I love that. I wish I could have that handbag." "If I could only dress like her." "If I only had that confidence to speak up in the meeting."

Or, if a colleague spoke up and said something "dumb" (that my in-the-box, calculated self would never have the courage to say in order to feel safe), I might think, "Oh my gosh, I can't believe she said that." My whole life was lived in this "palace" of judgment and criticism because I felt insecure in who I really was.

Because I wasn't being my true Self, the gap was widening between my external-world self and how I really felt inside. I had no clue that the challenges I started to face in my life were related to the widening gap. I wasn't speaking up for myself, finding my voice, or letting myself truly feel what needed to be felt. Unbeknownst to me, this growing resistance was starting to express itself outwardly. Here is what I experienced:

I was ecstatic to be pregnant with my first child, a son. I was still rockin' heels at work, leading new-hire training at a pace of forty hours per week in addition to a forty-five-minute commute each way. I was dressing the part as I kept doing the most challenging job I could. Life was good because I had the job, and was going to have this perfect family. A perfect son. All seemed well because I was checking the boxes of my external equation. It didn't matter that I was exhausted at the end of the day and my feet were killing me.

At thirty-three weeks gestation, I developed severe abdominal pain. When I threw up on the way to work, I assumed it was due to my prenatal vitamin. But when the abdominal pain worsened, I reached out to my doctor, who told me to go to the emergency room, as it was after office hours and the pain was unbearable. In the ER, they monitored the baby, checked my blood pressure, and sent me home, but the pain continued to worsen. I went back the next day, then followed up with my obstetrician. She identified there was a slight possibility this could be an atypical presentation of HELLP syndrome.

HELLP syndrome is a rare autoimmune disorder. Essentially, it's a blood disorder that can have severe consequences to both mom and baby. My OB put me on bedrest, gave me a list of symptoms to be looking for, and said to be sure to take this seriously and go to the emergency room should my symptoms worsen.

They did. I declined quickly. My abdominal pain was so bad that I continued to vomit despite being on bedrest. Once in the emergency room, I began to lose consciousness. Next thing I knew, I was being sent in for an emergency Cesarean Section. At thirty-five weeks and one day gestation, it was time to have our son. This split-second decision to deliver him at this time saved my life.

My liver enzymes were so high and platelets so low, that my blood wasn't clotting after my C-section. No one recognized it at the time, but I continued to bleed internally.

After a day and a half in the intensive care unit, and nine blood transfusions, my doctor knew I needed to head back into surgery. My family could see the fear in her expert eyes as she "reassured" them before heading into surgery; she wasn't sure I would make it.

I was too sick to recognize what was going on, or to understand the trauma that my husband and family were facing at the thought of losing me. I barely got to see my newborn son for the first nine days after delivery because of my surgeries, transfusions, and recovery in intensive care. We didn't even have a name for him for the first several days because we were in survival mode.

I so badly wanted a complete family, in the way I envisioned it, with two kids—hopefully a son and daughter. I didn't take time to heal from my trauma, to pause and feel my feelings, but instead continued on in the only way I knew how. I "recovered" in the physical sense, became a mom on maternity leave, then returned to work, as I was expected to do. It all felt terrible. There wasn't enough time with my baby boy. I didn't want to go back to work; I wanted to be with him. I sure could have used some time in therapy to process everything that had happened, but I didn't go. I got back to the grind, back to the equation that I thought would work to make me feel whole.

Against the advice and pleas of my family, I sought to get pregnant again. I wanted to take this risk in a quest to create the ideal family I'd imagined. I was determined. This time, we understood my history and I fully trusted my OB. We developed a plan and proceeded with pregnancy number two. There was an approximate thirty percent chance of recurrence of HELLP, and if it does recur, it's usually not as severe.

Unfortunately, it did recur—even earlier and more seriously this time.

I remember getting a call from my doctor when I was thirty-two weeks pregnant. She asked when I last ate. Then she announced that since I had eaten breakfast around 8 a.m., we would be delivering our baby girl that day at 4 p.m. I thanked God that I'd be okay and, as I showered and packed for this scheduled delivery, I couldn't help but feel excited about meeting our daughter. She was delivered that day at 3 lb, 8 oz, and had a host of issues due to her prematurity. She was rushed to the neonatal intensive care unit to be intubated and proceeded to spend the next sixty-one days there. She couldn't eat, and couldn't keep her blood pressure or heart rate up. She was covered in IVs for liquid nutrition, electrodes, and face gear to help her breathe despite her partially-collapsed lung. This time, I was okay and I remember wondering what I had done wrong to cause this suffering for my newborn baby girl. I felt guilty for the few green teas and occasional sip of red wine I had.

The whispers had become shouts in the form of multiple health challenges and life becoming increasingly difficult for me. Yet I continued on and returned to work. I still wasn't listening to the whispers, shouts, yells, or cries. I did the only thing I knew how to do: keep going.

When we force ourselves forward in this way, we create internal resistance. It can result in a series of increasingly difficult events, strained relationships, rising stress and anxiety levels, or more anger and frustration. Left unchecked, it can lead to health issues, physical pain in the body, or what we perceive as "accidents" happening to us.

When we don't find that voice for ourselves, or process difficult experiences, our bodies cry out. These were my cries that had grown from subtle, but ignored, whispers. But I still didn't listen. And I share this with you so that you can have a different trajectory.

How do you know when you have resistance in your body and in your life? You feel it—and it doesn't feel good. It feels bad, negative, and unwanted. You want to ignore or push it away. It causes you to feel bad about yourself or judgmental about someone else. Resistance feels like generalized negativity.

The resistance can result in life forcing challenges upon us so that we finally wake up to another way, and proactively do the work.

You can start listening to those whispers that have, perhaps, grown into shouts, screams, and cries. If you've faced this significant difficulty in your life, recognize it's now in the past. You can learn from that experience, then let it go. You can make a conscious choice to do the work yourself.

Life doesn't have to start yelling at you, or crying out in desperation for you to listen. I will teach you how to listen to your voice instead of the collective external voice of expectation. This will allow you to take the first steps in becoming your authentic Self.

But first, let's look at one final stage in which you may find yourself.

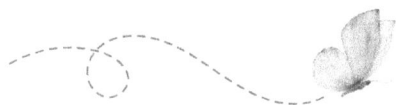

PART THREE

THE
FALL

Chapter Four

The Reckoning

In my life, I wasn't listening to the cries for change. I was so indoctrinated to the belief of the "right" way to approach my life that I kept showing up in the only way I knew how. I brushed off the traumatic experience of my children's births. Both times, I avoided feeling the gravity of it. Instead, I jumped into the responsibilities of motherhood and focused on getting my pre-baby body back. After what felt like a way-too-short maternity leave, I reluctantly returned to work because it was the only way I knew. Yet I felt such a deep longing to be with my kids. By not being there, I felt I was abandoning them—and my deepest desires. I had a pit in my stomach, felt sick about the thought of not being with them, and welled up with tears many days on my commute to the office.

I didn't listen to this feeling. Instead, I traveled forward on the only path I saw and knew.

On some level I felt that if I skipped a beat, had a hard day, or didn't continue, life would fall apart. I had to keep it together. It was as if I was standing on the edge of a cliff, and if I didn't work to constantly push away from the edge, I would fall deep into the unknown, feeling as if I would fall to my death. At the time I couldn't articulate any of this, but I was operating under the belief that if I didn't do it all, I would be nothing. Stuck in this black-and-white thinking pattern, I was driven by fear.

As a result of ignoring the whispers, which had turned to shouts, and stacking on others' expectations instead of my feelings, I was forced to face the reckoning.

The reckoning comes when you can no longer push against the edge of the cliff, and you start to fall. It's the point of no longer being able to ignore the yells from your life. It's the point where you fall to rock bottom. And I hit it.

First, the reckoning came in the form of additional struggles. Our daughter was born with a pre-melanoma that we had to get removed immediately. After spending the first two months of her life in the NICU, she underwent general anesthesia to have an extensive procedure performed on her scalp to remove the pre-cancer. I remember praying helplessly as her tiny body was rolled into surgery, and during the waiting period to get her biopsy results and prognosis. Desperate for her to be okay, I specifically pleaded, with tears in my eyes, "God, please do whatever it takes to keep our baby girl healthy. Please have her be cancer free and get all the margins. I'll even take it on if I have to." They got it all, thank God, and her prognosis was good.

Then my marriage started to struggle. Rocks started falling from beneath my feet as I neared the edge of the metaphorical cliff. I judged my husband for his lack of accountability, and for our financial struggles. My previously lucrative and "good" career was now in shambles. My boss was trying to push me out of the company, and finding every possible flaw in me to exploit. In doing this, she was touching on my deepest fears of unworthiness. I had never, in my life, felt such intense disapproval. If I still had the box I created to keep myself safe, I would have crawled into it, no question. But it had fallen with the rocks that were tumbling downward beneath my feet. I was in a downward spiral. We were barely getting by, barely keeping afloat. I was living my life tired, fatigued, exhausted, and feeling stuck and drained.

In the following months, my hairstylist suggested that I get a sore on my scalp checked out. I was healthy and knew it would be nothing, so I took my son to the doctor's appointment. He was about two-and-a-half-years old at the time, and I kept him entertained until my dermatologist walked in. He examined my scalp, asked a few questions, then sat down across from me. He took my hands in his, and shared that I had an aggressive form of Basal Cell Carcinoma. I had cancer. I had *cancer,* and in the exact same spot on my scalp as my daughter's pre-melanoma. Although he did his best to reassure me, tears welled up in my eyes. I couldn't hold back. I was scared and uncertain, deeply struggling with the idea that cancer could live in my body. I felt violated and afraid.

I had reached my reckoning and couldn't keep living this way.

This all had less to do with bad luck, and more to do with what I was creating in my life—and the fact that I needed to change.

Let me explain.

When we are living in this mode of survival, with ongoing stress, we are causing a whole host of issues inside ourselves. We are living in *catabolic energy.* Catabolic energy is necessary as it helps us hyper-focus on an immediate threat in front of us, so that we instinctively go into a flight, fight, or freeze response. When someone swerves into your lane on the road, or you are being physically attacked, you need the ability to subconsciously focus on the threat and have a cascade of instantaneous changes occur in your body. Your cells literally break down and release adrenaline and cortisol so that you can react without thinking. It's necessary for your survival, but it is detrimental if you stay in catabolic energy for too long.

I had been living my entire life in catabolic energy; many of us live the same way. You can recognize it by the way you are feeling. If you feel stressed, anxious, overwhelmed, tired, drained, angry, frustrated, or other "negative" emotions, you are in catabolic energy.

Another sure-fire way to know you are here is when you blame or are critical of yourself or others.

When you allow yourself to stay in this mode of survival, constantly pushing away from the edge of the cliff instead of healing from difficult life experiences, it only grows. What we resist, persists. I resisted the whispers, ignored the yells, and avoided the tough feelings. Much of my life had been spent in this catabolic place.

Catabolic energy, if left unchecked and unprocessed, leads to more problems. If you are familiar with the Universal Law of Attraction, it states that we attract more of what we think about and feel into our experience. Since I wasn't feeling good—living stressed, hyper-focused, driven by fear, and avoiding anything difficult—this brought more of the same experiences into my life. What I feared most was becoming my reality.

However, there is a solution.

This does not have to be your journey.

If you've experienced increasing difficulty and resistance in your life, that is enough information to recognize you are ready to make a change. You don't have to experience any more pain to choose another way.

I invite you to make the change yourself because if you don't, things will continue to spiral internally and externally. Difficult experiences will continue to show up in your life for two reasons. First, staying in this space of catabolic energy will attract more catabolic (challenging) experiences into your life. It's the Law of Attraction. Second, one of the main purposes in your life is to authentically move away from your negative, judgmental energy into another way of being. Since it's part of your journey anyway, why not choose a proactive approach instead of waiting for life to continue smacking you upside the head in an effort to teach you that there is another way?

If you feel you are teetering on the edge of the cliff and no longer have the strength to push back, like I did, this is your moment. You can decide if you will allow life to push you over the edge and hit rock bottom. Or, you can choose to stop pushing back and make a change.

Make the choice for yourself before it is made for you. It was made for me, and I'm still here to show you the other path. Use your agency and choose. I wish I had.

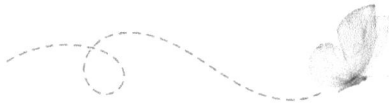

Chapter Five

The Shift

We are living in a stressful world where we believe we have to act a certain way in order to be loved and accepted. So making this "decision" to choose another way may seem difficult, if not impossible. In the following pages, we will uncover how you can choose a different path for yourself and your life. Together, we will walk forward into your Age of Beauty. Into a feeling of being whole, complete, and enough, just as you are. To be clear, this doesn't mean a switch will flip and you will be forever in this place, but with practice, it can absolutely become part of your life as it has mine.

My husband was tuned in to the sucky feelings of us being at rock bottom, and recognized there must be a better way. He had started going to therapy to save our marriage and came to me many times to gently ask if I would consider therapy too.

Before the fall to rock bottom, I would answer this question in my head with, "Me? No? I don't have any issues. I've been living this 'perfect' life with a 'perfect family' and the 'perfect career.'" This was the resistance. Even though my life was falling apart in front of my eyes, I politely declined.

He came to me week after week, sharing what he learned from his therapist and asking if I'd be interested in meeting with someone.

After the fall, I cracked open slightly. Being asked the same question—so nicely for so long—I started to wonder about the "why" behind it: Why did I keep saying no to him? Reluctantly, I stepped into a therapist's office, mostly to prove how "okay" I was.

Low and behold, my therapist, Connie, started to see and support me right away. And this came with uncovering a realization I had been hiding from and pushing away forever—that I was *not* okay. This opened the floodgates of feelings I'd been repressing.

I spent time crying in my room wondering what was wrong with me, going over the same questions in my mind. *Why wasn't I feeling closer to my kids? Why was my daughter born with pre-cancer on the top of her head? Why was it all so hard? Why me? How could cancer possibly be living in my body?*

The difference this time was that I allowed myself to pause, to feel the gravity of what I'd been through, rather than brushing it aside to move forward.

The unexpected beauty in the reckoning phase is that it cracks us open. We hit rock bottom and we crack. It's a shift that is both necessarily messy *and* beautiful.

When the floodgates of emotion first opened, it felt uncontrollable and overwhelming. I didn't recognize it at the time, but my constant attempts to control my outward experience failed; they cracked and a lifetime of repressed emotion came pouring out. I had to turn inward. It was the only way left and the only way out. I had to feel it all .

In each session with Connie, I learned something new. Each session, she would drag me through what felt like literal hell as she pulled me into the depths of feeling experiences from my past. Then I started to see this pattern of her moving me "from shit to light." Key to this was that I trusted her and felt safe. Each time she took me into depths of previously repressed emotion, I felt the hard feelings, and when I got to the other side, I felt lighter and more resilient. I could do this. After a while, I not only liked it, I craved it. This opened the door to a recognition that I both needed help *and* could rely on professionals to safely help me heal physically, mentally, and emotionally.

Over the next several years, I sought support from energy healers, clinical nutritionists, holistic health practitioners, and medical doctors. I listened to Oprah's *Super Soul* podcast religiously, and devoured other spiritual podcasts and self-help books. I spent hours consuming information during long drives for my job. I invested in a coach to help our daughter with her ADHD, a coach to resolve my "career crisis," and endless supplements to feel better in my body. I learned to meditate with the help of Gabrielle Bernstein, and eventually invested in my education to become a Certified Professional Coach.

I've invested over fifteen years and $200,000 in this quest to find another way. And now, I will share my learnings with you in a way that doesn't require anywhere near that amount of time or financial investment.

This next section will walk you, step-by-step, through how to tune into your true beauty as a woman. Much of this information will feel new, yet strangely familiar. This is because you will be brought back to the Truth of who you are, and who you always were.

You will discover the You that was, somehow, lost along the way, through the tapestry of societal expectation.

The alternative, of course, is to stay the course. Keep doing what you are doing. Keep relying on Botox and expensive skincare. Save up for the laser procedure, or the new handbag to ease the burden. Keep focusing on anti-aging in all ways you can. You know that this path provides boosts of "confidence," yet leaves the underlying sense of lack unaddressed. On this path, you can expect life will continue to whisper, yell, or scream at you to change.

Change doesn't mean you need to stop enjoying all the wonderful technologies and advancements we have available to us to help us feel our best. Keep being you. Keep rockin' with your bad self. Just know that when you consciously choose to invest in yourself, by learning and practicing the steps outlined in this next section and workbook, you will be on your way to stepping into your unique Age of Beauty.

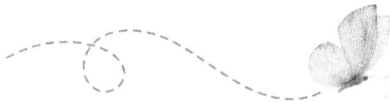

Here we go!

PART FOUR

THE DEPTH

Chapter Six

Finding YOU-th

T he first thing you get to do is find your YOU-th. And it doesn't have to come in the form of the latest expensive anti-aging cream or energy supplement. You get to do this by owning your energy. Remember how catabolic energy drains and exhausts us, leaving us feeling depleted and tired? We know we are in it if we are feeling anxious, isolated, alone, afraid, worried, or run down. If we are comparing ourselves to others, judging situations and ourselves, we are in catabolic energy. When we are in this energy for an extended period of time, it leaves cortisol and adrenaline running through our veins. The prolonged state is not only tied to a whole host of health issues but also accelerates our aging process, leaving us not feeling as youthful or beautiful.

This is the way that many of us operate—on default.

OWN YOUR ENERGY

There is a whole new way of looking at and operating through a "higher" energy called *anabolic energy*. Anabolic energy is the energy that heals, allows us to relax and unwind, and to see our world from a broader perspective. It makes us feel good, feel better. When we are in it, not only do we have good-feeling hormones like dopamine and serotonin running through our bodies, but our body digests, heals, and repairs itself as it is designed to.

Anabolic energy isn't an energy that happens by chance due to our external world. We actually get to choose it. Yes, we can acknowledge that there are a lot of challenges in the world. But there is also a lot of good. It depends on how we perceive it. Either way, we are at a place of choosing, which means we are no longer "victims" to our external circumstances.

You get to choose how you respond in every single situation. With practice, anabolic energy is an energetic state you can learn to live in.

Having fun slows down your biological clock and widens the gap between your numerical, or chronological, and biological age. Fun is a quick creator of anabolic energy. When you choose to act like the kid you were, or the kid you deserved to be (but maybe didn't get to fully experience because of the expectations placed upon you), you are creating high-vibe energy. You have a choice to be and do something supportive for yourself. You can skip. You can have fun. You can laugh more. You can prioritize time off, relaxation, and friends over work.

I choose to act like a kid when I hold my daughter's hand and skip through the neighborhood. Our neighbors may think I'm crazy, but I'm laughing and connecting with my daughter and living in my joy. I literally cannot feel stressed, anxious, or bad while skipping.

Another practice to boost my energy—that I struggled with initially, and eventually mastered—was the art of dialing back my efforts at work. Due to fear and imposter syndrome, I'd always given 110% at work, to ensure I would be protected by my perfection. Giving 110% felt like my armor against anyone who may criticize or judge my work, or me. I experimented with taking more time to reply to an email instead of responding immediately, with my heart racing, to ensure I looked "on top of things". I asked for a demotion and gladly took it when a position opened up. I continued to take time during the day for self-care, including sneaking away for a haircut or to get my nails done. And instead of listening to the shameful voice that was worried I'd get caught, I consciously recognized that everyone needs a break, and breathed my way through it. I began blocking my calendar for personal reasons, like picking up the kids from the bus everyday. And I'm pleased to report, my job became more enjoyable and energizing. Not only was I putting in less time and effort (maybe 80%), but I had more energy for work when I came back to it after building more time for me into my day. Eventually, I learned to set boundaries for myself versus letting my every move be controlled by an infinite number of imagined expectations. Surprisingly, no one noticed the change in effort or my shifting priority of work; I was still getting great reviews, completing my work, and receiving genuine, positive feedback from others. When we set boundaries for ourselves, everyone wins.

If you are feeling hesitant, maybe wondering if this seems childish or unfeasible with your work demands, let's reframe it.

It's wonderful when you can learn to prioritize fun and enjoyment first in your day because it starts you off in a higher energy that sets the tone for the rest of your day. Everything will flow more easily, feel more doable, and be more enjoyable because you are approaching it from a higher energy and perspective. Specifically, savoring your favorite latte, lighting a candle, going for a walk or taking time to smile or laugh will help you better enjoy this life and show up more fully at work. It's a win-win.

Perhaps you remember being a young girl playing freely, fully in the present moment, laughing, smiling, skipping, and being unattached to outcomes. Or, if this wasn't your experience, you may have observed it in young children and puppies who innately live in their joy of expression, in the fullness of life. They are close to the reality of who they are, as unique and unlimited beings. Nothing is off the table in terms of creativity or expression. They are attuned to their true Selves, and connected to everyone around them without judgment or comparison, just observation and curiosity.

Prioritize fun and joy in your day. And I encourage you to do it first. Don't let it wait until your tasks and "To-Dos" for the day are done. If you do, you will probably be too tired to prioritize it, and the benefit of it will be diminished. If you raise your vibe at the end of the day, you only have a short time to enjoy it before you go to bed. Why not start earlier, and prioritize yourself and your joy first?

The practices I use to start my day in joy are to, upon first waking up, think of three things I'm grateful for and one thing I will let go of (that is no longer serving me). This is a powerful way to change the narrative of my day as compared to the usual voice of "Oh man, I'm so tired," "Ugh, I have so much to do today," or my heart racing because I hit snooze one too many times and my mind starts running through all that I have to do for the day and the time each will take—feeling immediately overwhelmed.

Head over to the workbook to identify feasible ways you can choose your energy, prioritize fun and joy, and start your day in a high-vibe state.

YOU ARE NOT YOUR AGE

A second principle I want to introduce to you is that you are not your age.

You are your energy.

You know those people who walk into the room and instantly capture your attention and the attention of others? They have a radiance about them, something captivating. What you may not recognize is that this is less about their age, and more about their energy. And you can harness this for yourself in your desire to feel more youthful.

These people carry excitement, vibrance, and radiance. Simply put, they are living in a higher, more anabolic energy. Jean Ketcham, author and founder of the online community *Aging but Dangerous,* embodies this beauti- fully. Eighty-four-years-old and full of energy, she carries herself with her head held high, owns who she is, and is full of life. She is beautiful as a result of this!

Conversely, you've seen a teenage girl slumped over her phone, probably subconsciously comparing herself to others on social media, and feeling "less than." She is clearly lacking confidence and presence. Her head is down. Her eyes are tired. She has all the youth one could hope for, but isn't tapping into or harnessing the energy available to her. She may not appear beautiful in your eyes, despite her youth, because she isn't stepping into her strength and power. She isn't consciously choosing her energy and, therefore, doesn't have that youthful glow.

You can learn to recognize and notice your energy. When you choose a higher, more anabolic energy, you can slow down the aging process. Remember, you are not your age. You are your energy.

FIND YOU

Another way to find more youth in your life is to find YOU. If you are struggling to know who you are at this point, because you've committed your life to focusing on others' needs, that's okay. I was there too, operating under the tapestry of life and society for so long. Before the fall, my life was "in order" and all the pieces fit perfectly together because I oversaw and controlled the construction of it. After the fall, I recall sitting in my therapist Connie's office, feeling like the puzzle of my life had been thrown up in the air and destroyed. There were a million pieces flying around and I didn't know where they were going to land or what the picture of my life would look like. It was a scary and unsettling feeling because I had no sense of who I truly was. I had no clue what I wanted or how I could start a new life and have it come together into anything recognizable.

If you're feeling this, it's okay and it's normal. Your life can, and will, be reconstructed, piece by piece. One of the first ways to do this is to notice if the decisions you make throughout your day, no matter how big or small, feel good to you, or not. Are you making your choice based on what you want, or because you feel like you "should?" This will, decision by decision, allow you to start finding yourself.

When you're considering taking that new job, for example, make your decision based on what feels good to you. Ask yourself the following questions:

Does it excite and elevate you?

Are you choosing to take it out of trust that it will work out, and know that if it doesn't, you will still be okay?

Or, are you choosing to stay because you are afraid of the unknown, or afraid others might judge you for following your desire?

Are you choosing from fear and lack?

You will learn to notice that when you make choices out of opportunity, or higher anabolic energy, you will be guided more often to this energy, and find your True Self faster than if you let fear run the show.

When I am deciding whether to exercise in the morning, I ask myself how the decision feels. An anabolic choice feels energizing, like I am prioritizing my self care, and know this will be a good start to my day. It doesn't matter if one day I decide to get up and work out, and the next day I decide to sleep in and rest. Based on how it feels to me, I know which option is best for me on any given day.

Conversely, a catabolic decision, one made out of fear, might sound like, "I am tired, and don't want to, but I really should work out." It's more forced than in flow. On days where it's forced, I either shift my energy or, if I'm unable to do that, I skip the workout altogether. Start to make decisions and challenge the status quo by recognizing whether you're choosing out of high-vibe, good feeling energy, or fear and lack. Start to choose more of what you do want, and less of what you do not want. Tune into how you feel. Check in with your heart and gut for guidance, and you will become increasingly more aligned with who you are, and what you want. And you will be in a higher-vibe, more YOU-thful energy.

Eventually, after making more and more choices that feel good to you, you will learn to recognize who you are. You will have turned inward to notice what you want, as opposed to what others expect. You will learn to express your wishes and wants, and recognize that doing so wasn't as scary as you thought. The world is not black and white—either focus on yourself or others. When you prioritize yourself, and show up in your authentic expression, the world adapts and adjusts. You get to be yourself, and own your YOU-th. It's a beautiful unfolding.

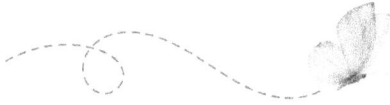

Chapter Seven

Inner Beauty and Radiance

HAPPY GIRLS ARE THE PRETTIEST GIRLS

You've probably heard Audrey Hepburn's words, "happy girls are the prettiest girls." When we are truly happy and joyful in our journey, we develop an inner radiance, beauty, and excitement that exudes from us. And it just so happens that others notice it too. We smile more. Remember what we said about you not being your age? You are actually your energy. It's so true.

When you tap into joy, happiness, and completeness, you are at the highest levels of anabolic energy. Not only do you appear more radiant to others, but you have greater enjoyment of the whole ride of life. And, as an added bonus, you slow down your biological clock. You truly feel more youthful in your body because you are focused on the feeling within.

While happiness may not be a pinnacle, or state, that you ever fully reach, you can absolutely work on your "happierness"—a term coined by Oprah and Arthur Brooks. You can create moments of feeling happy by recognizing that you can choose your default state—happy or unhappy—in any moment. You actually have a choice on how you let life impact you, as opposed to being at its mercy with a belief that, "Once I have _____, then I will be happy."

The truth is that when you wait for something in your external environment to change in order to be happy, you are in an inherent state of lack. For example, if you subconsciously believe that our political landscape, your work environment, or your body shape, needs to change in order to be happy, then you are, by definition, unhappy at this moment. It sets up and perpetuates an endless cycle of less-than.

I operated in a state of lack for the first half of my life. I was striving, and working, and hustling with the hope that the sacrifice of today would create the happiness of tomorrow. I learned, after banging my head against the wall for years, that I could no longer push, control, and achieve my way into happiness. I had to learn to choose it for myself and my life, through practice, in the here and now. For me, it meant slowing down enough to relish in the moments of snuggling my kids, or taking a moment to sit with and pet our dogs before starting my day. It has come from learning to let go of difficult situations in an attempt to look at them through a lens of understanding instead of anger and resentment.

You, too, can lean into small moments throughout your day that bring you true happiness, and recognize that you have a choice in how you let something undesirable impact you. Remember, when you own your happiness, you will feel more radiant.

MIRROR MIRROR ON THE WALL

A pivotal experience shaped my belief that there is something deeper, an essence beyond words, in each of us. After showing some lethargic tendencies, we received the news that our six-year-old hunting dog, Gage, had lung cancer that had metastasized throughout his body. We didn't have much time left with him, and my husband was distraught about the thought of losing such a wonderful companion who had brought him so much joy.

We did our best to maximize our time with him, through tears, special bites of steak, and lots of hugs. When it was time to put him down, when he was no longer walking or eating, our veterinarian came to our home. She walked us through what to expect during her visit, and I listened intently while my husband held back tears. He didn't have it in him to be physically in the room when Gage passed on, so I snuggled up close to our beloved dog, letting him know how much I loved him, and gazed deeply into his eyes as I stroked his ears.

After our vet administered the second shot, I recall looking at Gage and wondering when he'd leave us. And when he did, I knew the instant it happened, even before the vet confirmed his passing. I saw the light and spark in his eyes fade to darkness, and felt a simultaneous surge of energy pass upward through my hand.

Take a moment to think about the words you use to describe the intangible essence of a person, the core of their being that is almost beyond words. It's the part of them that feels eternal and timeless, that connects them to something greater than themselves. It's the part of them that expresses love, compassion, empathy, and spirituality. For me, this word is *soul*. Perhaps your word is spirit, core, consciousness, or essence. No matter the word, it's part of every being, and it's part of you.

A powerful technique I learned from Louise Hay—author, speaker, healer, teacher, and artist—is an exercise you can use daily in the mirror to connect with this more soulful, deeper essence of who you are.

Instead of your default tendency to focus on your flaws, try gazing into your eyes in your reflection to connect with the deep, spiritual side of You. It's the part of you that has an inner light and radiance; a spark. It's the part of you that is eternal, naturally whole and complete. Here, there is nothing to judge, because you are present and connected.

If you feel called, as you continue to gaze into your eyes, say to yourself the words, "I love you." Repeat them several times. At first, you may feel awkward and disconnected from the purpose of the exercise. Eventually, with practice, you will begin to sense there is another part of you beyond this physical form. You'll remember, more often, that there is a deeper essence to you, a beauty beyond your physical form, that when nurtured will create more inner assuredness and outward radiance.

RELATIONSHIP WITH FEAR

It might sound weird, but it's time to develop a deeper relationship with fear.

Understanding fear in your life, and how it shows up, is a key skill. You probably already know what it feels like to be afraid, worried, scared, or uncertain but understanding how it drives your actions is a whole other level. We will get to more in-depth ways to release fear's grip on your life later, but for now, just know that the more you recognize it, the less hold it has on you. The first step in any journey is the awareness of what you are truly feeling.

It's easiest—and often our default tendency—to avoid difficult emotions, and yet it is through our sheer resistance to, and avoidance of, these situations that they persist and continue to show up in our lives. Instead of avoiding, pretending it doesn't exist, or ignoring it, it's time to call it out. When you notice fear showing up, you can acknowledge you are feeling anxious, worried, or afraid, then say to yourself, "Oops, I must be choosing out of fear again, but I don't have to." Then, you can choose to focus on something else, a more loving perspective of the same situation. This will release the emotional hold on you. Remember, this is a choice you get to make.

The more you recognize, own, and accept your current state of fear, the better able you will be to let it go. Many of my clients want to learn to "let go" but have no clue where to start. This is a beautiful place to start. You see, when we avoid something, we are pushing against it, and our sheer resistance to it will make it persist. According to Carl Jung, "What you resist not only persists, but will grow in size."

A client of mine who owns a medical practice came to me due to some disrespectful behavior from her employees. When we first started working together she didn't realize that because she was afraid of potential criticism of the current culture, she didn't solicit feedback from others, or address situations head on. She feared appearing confrontational and unapproachable and wanted to be well liked and well respected. What resulted for her team was a feeling of confusion, uncertainty about where they stood, and resultant chatter. Despite her best efforts, the culture had become toxic.

Through our work together, she learned to face difficult patients in her practice head on, not defensively, but with open curiosity. Her employees observed this and began following suit. She did the same with her team, calling out challenges and asking for their input and ideas. Within our first few months of working together, she was overjoyed by the conversation she overheard in the breakroom. One of her employees stated that the whole energy of the practice had changed! She couldn't put a finger on it, but she knew it felt better. Another employee chimed in with, "I feel it too." Even more important was how my client felt after facing a situation head on. Instead of letting a difficult conversation play out in her mind in an infinite number of ways, she asked the questions she needed to ask to be clear on what was really happening, then felt confident in her ability to make more informed decisions.

It was so empowering to witness her, in a few short months, shift her way of showing up by facing fears head on, with curiosity, instead of subconsciously avoiding them for fear of what she might learn, or of judgment from others.

Acceptance is about recognizing and owning where you are. In that awareness you can choose to stop pushing so hard. You can begin to trust that if life is pushing you in a certain direction, even if it is toward the edge of the cliff; there is a reason—and that you will be okay. You can let go and trust that even if you do fall, the landing will be softer than expected. Perhaps instead of deadly terrain, there are supportive clouds below you can't see from your vantage point. And when you fall, you will get back up again. It's the fall that helps us get closer to our true Selves, finally free from the fear that has been running the show for so long.

Head over to the workbook and start this week to identify ways to feel happier, along with ways to begin accepting that you truly are greater and more beautiful than you currently accept yourself to be. You will also learn ways to create a different relationship with the things you are most afraid of in a journey to learning your true strength and resilience. It isn't about mastering fear, as it will always be present to some degree, but rather developing a deeper relationship with it to learn your deeper beauty within.

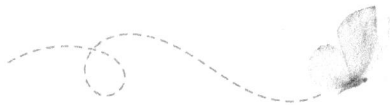

Chapter Eight

From Wellness to Wholeness

In many ways the "wellness" industry feels like an updated, more socially acceptable word to describe the beauty industry. It still includes hefty diet, exercise, and supplement trends in an effort to become something more or different than who you are now. There is nothing inherently wrong with these offerings, yet I imagine you desire to take advantage of both the latest wellness trends, *and* to feel whole and complete in the woman you are already. You can, by following these three steps.

RAISE YOUR VIBE

The first way to step into the fullness and wholeness of who you are is to raise your vibe by doing something daily that centers and grounds you. It's a bit of a paradox, but when we feel grounded and safe in who we are, we get to more fully experience the highs of life. Some practices to consider include: a morning gratitude practice, getting out in nature, committing to not checking your phone for the first forty-five minutes after you wake up, meditating, slowing your breath, or practicing yoga. The options are endless, and as you decide how you will raise your daily vibe, be sure to choose something that takes minimal time and that you can truly develop into a daily practice. It has to be achievable, even on days you feel short on time.

As you commit to this new practice in your life, take it in your stride. You will certainly miss days—and that is okay. If you judge yourself, you will immediately lose any feel-good energy, and will drop right back into catabolic energy. Instead, you can acknowledge the miss, and come up with a plan that allows you to resume the practice which, of course, can evolve and change as you do. What is most important is that you are consistently taking a moment of time each day to prioritize your own centering and wellbeing.

REFRAME YOUR PAST

This can be a difficult one, as our pasts inherently shape who we are today. And yet, many women I work with expect their past mistakes and missteps to be part of their future. It's as though the past has been branded on them, and is expected to show up again and again. Let me explain.

One of the most difficult times in my life was when I was working at a company I'd been with for almost ten years. I had a new boss, and she found every possible flaw in me, from what and where I expensed, to what times I ate meals. She questioned my every move. She was out to get me, and I could feel it. It caught me completely off guard, as I'd had a great experience up until that point, had been promoted several times and felt highly supported. What I didn't put together was that my division was projected to do better than the one she had a background in, and this was a professional and personal threat to her.

She made my life a living hell by tracking my where-abouts and calling multiple times per day to question my interactions with customers and colleagues. She even got to the point of reporting me to Human Resources, on two separate occasions, for expenses I had made that had been expensed (and approved) by prior managers multiple times before. When I tried to explain myself to her, she labeled me as "uncooperative and disrespectful." When I offered to correct it, and pay out of pocket, she wouldn't allow it, saying, "The damage of your dishonesty has already been done." When I asked around to see if others on my team were having the same experience, she called me "conniving and manipulative." I felt like I couldn't win, no matter what I did. I started to question myself, my integrity, my worth at the company I thought I knew and trusted.

I spent nights at home crying to my husband, feeling so scared about being fired and not knowing what else to do, as I had been with that company most of my career. I recall not sleeping well, feeling like I had to act "perfectly" at all times to avoid any other reports to HR. When I was approached by one of the senior leaders to be promoted to his team, which would have been my biggest promotion yet, she went out of her way to ruin that opportunity for me by claiming I was unreliable, unfit, and dishonest.

The stress I was under became so great that I fell short of breath before answering her phone calls, and stayed stuck in my mind for endless hours, playing out "what if" scenarios for every step I made, afraid of how she would respond.

I knew I had to get out, as I couldn't see any other path forward and, reluctantly, started looking for a new job. Thankfully, I quickly got a great position outside the company. Even though it paid substantially less, I have never looked back.

If I let it, this experience could live in my mind indefinitely, and anytime I recall it, bring me immediately back to this place of imposter, not enough, something-is-wrong-with-me, energy. Or, I could reframe my past.

So, I have.

I now look upon this time with gratitude for all I learned. I learned that when someone is treating me horribly, I still have control of how I respond. Even though the experience sucked, I showed up for myself and did what I had to for my financial future. I protected myself. I can acknowledge the great career I had there, instead of letting the bitterness of one experience define me. I now appreciate that all the worthlessness I felt was never about me, but rather about her not liking me. I forgive her because, even though I believe she was capable of being more kind, she was doing the best she knew how. I know that this past only exists in my mind. It's no longer here, and when I look upon it for its learning, or let it go, it no longer controls me.

You, too, can reframe your past with practice—and let me tell you, it is a beautiful and freeing experience. Head over to the workbook to do this for yourself in your own life. Once complete, be sure to allow yourself to feel the changed energy around the situation. You can come back to this exercise any time you are struggling with a past experience.

BEYOND BEAUTY

This is the stage where you learn to trust your intuition, inner knowing, higher Self, or soul. It's the part of you that may have laid dormant much of your life, but has always been there, waiting for you to invite it in. Waiting for you to quiet the external focus, the hustle and grind, to pause and to check in on it. As you do, you will learn not only to hear or know what this part of you is saying, but also learn to trust this guidance. It's a state of alignment, and when you are in an aligned place, you are always being guided in the best direction for yourself.

We all desire to feel beautiful, particularly as we age. And beneath that desire to feel beautiful is a desire to feel loved and accepted, wholly, as we are. So, how do we move beyond the latest diet, exercise, or beauty trend to feeling truly whole and complete as women?

Since most of our beauty and wellness industry has been focused on external indicators of "beauty," it's no wonder that the majority of advances have come in the form of physical improvement, through optimized nutrition, supplementation, exercise, and the latest med-spa treatment or cream. And these advancements have done just that—helped us to advance how we feel about ourselves as we age.

To move from wellness to wholeness, however, we also need to address our mental, emotional, and spiritual wellness. If you feel overwhelmed about how to do this at the moment, don't worry. We can take this piece by piece, by learning to recognize, prioritize, and support our wellness, moment to moment, day to day. As we do, we will feel more whole in who we are, because we haven't left any parts of us behind in our quest to feel physically and socially dialed in. So, how do we do this?

To move beyond the wellness you have committed to, and into wholeness, you need to start turning inward. Your mental, emotional, and spiritual wellbeing are all "inside jobs." You no longer need to look outward to compare your outfit, or weight, to another woman or your younger self. Instead, you can use yourself as a barometer: "How do I feel today compared to how I felt yesterday?" "Am I comfortable in the clothes I'm wearing?" "Did I move my body in a way that felt good today?"

The simplest way to identify your inner state is to recognize whether you feel predominantly good or bad in a given moment. If it's good, keep going. Enjoy the moment, and also consider what it is—specifically about you—that has helped to create that good-feeling vibe.

Conversely, if you're not feeling good, it's an indicator that your emotional, mental, or spiritual energy is off. Acknowledge it without judgment, then consider what needs to happen in order for you to feel better.

Then listen. You will be guided. You will know when you are tapped into the inner voice when it feels peaceful, calm, and certain. It tends to be clear, consistent, and kind, like it's coming from a loving place.

When I'm feeling overwhelmed by work, my heart racing with endless "to-dos," I stop to notice it, then ask, "What do I need right now to get back into balance?" Often an idea pops into my head—to go outside for a walk, take a nap, or take time to meditate—and I listen to it. In the past, I may have brushed off this still, quiet, inner voice in the name of completing the email, or pushing toward a deadline. But now, I listen in and act. In taking this action, I discovered that when I take the time I need for self-care in the moment, I come back to work feeling refreshed, with new energy and perspective.

At other times when I feel off and ask this same question, I learn that I need to allow myself to feel the feelings of the "bad" state. So I do. I will get up from my desk, walk out to my car or over to the couch, and allow myself to feel the full gravity of my heart racing in my chest, how completely overwhelmed I am, how sad and unmotivated I feel, or whatever else has risen to the surface. I often cry, hunch over, and allow myself to fully feel the feeling. For a few minutes I let it all out. And then, surprisingly, it's cleared.

What I used to resist no longer persists because I've addressed and allowed it to move through me. This is a paradoxical way to nurture your inner state by allowing the "bad" energy to move through you, but it works.

Remember, you have everything you need within you to feel whole and complete in the woman you are. You have the power to raise your vibe, to reframe your past in such a way that it no longer controls or defines you, and to grow beyond your external beauty by focusing inward on your spiritual, mental, and emotional wellbeing. This is how you move, moment to moment, into ultimate wholeness. From wellness to wholeness.

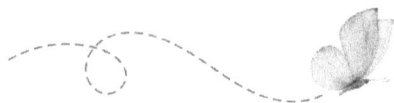

Chapter Nine

Confidence

M uch like the beauty industry has focused on our external look, confidence too often comes from how we look and, therefore, feel about ourselves from a body-image or external standpoint. As we age, this "ideal image" becomes fleeting and harder to maintain. We can have it in a given moment when someone pays us attention or a compliment, but lose it the next because, by definition, it is coming from how others react to and accept us, or how we stack up relative to others.

Think back to a time when you used to be "more confident." Were you just more accepted by others for who you were previously, more compliant, hard working, or youthful? True confidence is an inside job. It's not about regaining what you once had, but rather growing it from the inside, so that it can radiate outward. Then it can exude through you, and attract even more goodness into your life.

Here's the first step.

GROW YOUR CONFIDENCE

Gaining real confidence means accessing your true, deep sense of value beyond what shows up as a fleeting boost. It requires you to develop trust and kindness toward yourself, to grow that sense of self-love and, perhaps for the first time, fuel your body, mind, and spirit in a whole new way. Instead of comparing yourself to another woman, how you used to look, or what you feel you "should" look like at your age, start to view your body as a vehicle that allows you to love, express yourself, and experience all of the wonder and beauty of this life. You get to enjoy and spread love in the world, and your body allows you to do that. You get to have fun. You get to travel. You get to have all these passions and experiences at your fingertips through a committed, yet simple, inner voice reframe.

Remember that your body is not of your creation. Regardless of your spiritual beliefs, we all are uniquely different, and you were created as you are to be essentially perfect. You are beautiful. You are complete as is. Nothing has to physically change in order for you to recognize and accept this about yourself.

Making the choice to love yourself is the ultimate act of confidence. You're going to be inherently different from every other woman and person in this world because you are uniquely you. The whole idea of comparing and contrasting is a futile exercise. It's never going to work in a long-term, sustainable way. We are never going to be the tallest, thinnest, have the most flowy hair, have the best curls, the longest eyelashes, all the time. External beauty is fleeting. It's just not possible. There's always going to be someone who is different and uniquely beautiful in her own light.

There is a higher knowing, a higher perspective, that comes when you can love and look at yourself in such a way that you know and trust you are whole and complete as you are. Instead of focusing on the little confidence boosters that come with fixing a flaw, or sizing yourself up relative to someone else, you can shift your perspective to something you genuinely love or appreciate about your body.

I have a huge scar that runs from my left shoulder to my elbow, and covers the two rods, and seventeen pins that reconstructed my arm after a traumatic arm break while skiing. When my doctor unwrapped the bandages from my arm for the first time after surgery, I couldn't believe what I saw. The scar was so significant, unsightly, and jarring to look at. My self-confidence took a huge hit. I was a perfectionist in many ways and this scar represented the death of any future hope of being "perfect."

I never felt perfect in the first place, but I strove for it relentlessly, thanks to a deep fear of inadequacy. As I gazed at my arm, this part of me died. Part of my ego died along with the hope of being able to look a certain way. That led to the death of feeling a certain way about myself. I could no longer hide my internal feelings of being flawed through striving. My flaws were now out in the world for everyone to see.

When I look back honestly on how I felt about myself and my body before this accident, I realize I never felt truly beautiful anyway. There was always something that held me back from seeing myself as whole, complete, and perfect just as I was. At times it was my unruly curls, then the C-section scars. Before that, it was the scar on top of my head after my basal cell carcinoma had been removed that created a "unicorn horn"—a tuft of hair—growing back over a golf-ball-sized area on my scalp that had been removed and reconstructed.

There has always been some part of me that I noticed and judged.

I know now I had been spending all this time focused on the negative when, really, my true beauty was always there. Seeing myself as I am today, perfectly imperfect, doesn't mean those old scars are gone. The truth is, I made a choice to focus on that one flaw and ignore the perfect, beautiful creation that I was. Alternatively, I could choose all the things I genuinely love and appreciate about myself and that I am grateful for. My health.

My family. My power. My voice. My kindness. The radiance in my eyes. My energy. There is so much more.

To move toward a deeper level of self love that goes beyond an occasional, comparative confidence boost, usually inspired by an external change, remember that beauty is in the eyes of the beholder. You are the eyes for which you see and judge your own beauty. Let those eyes be kind and loving instead of critical and harsh. In other words, own your power to love and appreciate your own beauty, instead of giving it away to the eyes of others at the expense of knowing yourself and your beauty more deeply. There is a deep level of self-love that transcends external confidence—and it comes with making a decision to listen more to the kind, loving voice instead of the fearful, lacking one.

The way I tap into this higher knowledge is to tune in and ask the universe. I ask my soul—my higher wisdom—things like, "I'm tired today. Is this still a good day to work out?" and I listen. Sometimes that answer is yes, and it's guiding me to go out there to move my body because something good is going to come from it. And other times it says, "No. It's okay to rest today." And I listen to that loving, guiding, certain voice that comes in after I ask questions, instead of the fearful voice that told me I *should* workout, because I'm lazy if I don't, or I need to do it in order to stay fit. This loving voice gives a small boost of true confidence, but in a lasting way. And it's always there. I can access it and invite it in at any point.

Oftentimes, the women I work with want to regain the confidence they had in their twenties, but the truth is, that version of themselves is gone. And, if you're being fully honest with yourself, you probably didn't feel all that confident then, either. You may have had it "all together" from the lens of looking back on your thinner frame, higher energy, and thicker hair, but let's face it: you were looking toward other women that you somehow felt were more than you, while you felt less than, perhaps wanting more money in order to be "successful", or that you wouldn't be complete until you found "the one." You weren't fully appreciating the woman you were then, much like you aren't fully appreciating the woman you are now. And yet, it's certain that one day you'll look back on this time fondly, wishing you would have appreciated the beauty of today. Your beauty of today.

What's stopping you from doing that now? It only requires a shift in perspective. Confidence is an inside job, and shifting from external focus to inner beauty makes all the difference. You can ignore these words and keep reading, or you can declare to yourself right now, perhaps in the mirror, that from this day forward you will see yourself in a more loving light. You will choose to focus on your gifts and strengths instead of shortcomings and flaws. When you mess up (because you will), you'll forgive your thoughts. You'll come back to a more loving way to view yourself, through every age and stage of life. This is where deep, lasting, true confidence is born.

And you get to claim this for your life.

UNDERSTAND YOUR VALUE(S)

Another important piece to feeling more confident is to understand what you value most. According to Dr. Wayne Dyer in his documentary *The Shift*, most women maintain the values of family, independence, career, fitting in, and attractiveness (Dyer 2009). You can see the inherent conflict in some of these. First off, family, career, fitting in and attractiveness are all based on others' needs and expectations of us. Each one is outwardly focused. Your boss and colleagues define your work success. Your family requires your constant consideration and giving. Your "fitting in" and level of "attractiveness" are based on how others perceive and react to you. Yet independence is there too. You yearn to be more yourself, more authentically you in a world that you've given your power away to. And there is an inherent value conflict in this.

Knowing that you want to find more of your voice, independence, and true value, let's determine what it is, at this stage in your life, that matters most to you. Not only will this give you more clarity in who you are, being clear on what you value will give you the framework you need to make decisions in your life.

Once you identify your top three-to-five values in the workbook, and know them with certainty, you get to make decisions that align with who you truly are. For

81

example, my values are: love, joy, freedom, and connection. The last one used to be "belonging," but then I recognized that, too, was giving my power away to those who decided (not myself) whether I "belonged" or not. Instead, I chose "connection." I know in my heart when I make a meaningful connection to someone. So, if I get a job opportunity in an industry I don't love, that pays a lot of money, and comes with a set schedule, it might not be the right fit for me because I value freedom and joy so much. Yet I also value connection, so I need to consider the culture there, to decide if that value could be fulfilled. By understanding your values, you'll be better able to make decisions in your life that support you from a true, deep, standpoint of self-worth and confidence.

This clarity in values can allow you to filter a decision, no matter how large or seemingly insignificant, through this lens. This can allow you to decide quickly and with clarity what is for you and what is not. Many women I work with desire to make decisions then move on and let them go. This is a sure-fire way to get there.

YOU ARE NOT THE VOICE INSIDE YOUR HEAD

Have you ever heard of the gremlin voice? I first heard that term in my iPEC coaching program. It can go by many names, but essentially, it's the voice inside your head that tells you that you are not enough in some way.

Every single one of us has this voice, and more often than not, we listen to it. When we listen to and believe this voice, we give it unearned power that negatively impacts our confidence and self-worth. Instead, we can choose to notice it and handle it in a different way. We can reframe that voice for ourselves, recognizing that it is a small part—not all—of us, and it is not speaking the truth.

This voice was initially created as a form of protection—to keep you safe. This can be confusing because it feels predominantly negative. Perhaps your voice encouraged you to get better grades so your parents wouldn't get mad at you, or work harder so you could make the team. This same gremlin voice that now can cause you so much suffering, was initially helping you to fit in, which is a core human need. We are wired for connection, so it's not all bad. It just is an outdated form of protection that is likely no longer serving you.

Here is what my gremlin sounds like:

Keep going. It doesn't matter that you're tired.

You have to respond to that email before bed, or they'll think you're slacking.

You better say yes to that project if you want to be considered for any promotions in your future.

You better go to the soccer game, even though you aren't feeling well.

Try harder.

Your wrinkles are getting bad.

The cellulite on your legs is gross.

Better hurry and pick up before your friends get here. You don't want to look like a slob.

You should feel guilty for not working as hard today.

The underlying message of my gremlin has been one of needing to hustle for my worth. As if I'm somehow not loveable, not enough, to just be me. This gremlin voice drove me to work so hard, to be a perfectionist, to give 110%. It helped me overachieve in every area of life but, ultimately, led to my burnout and health issues.

There is another, more loving, voice inside—the voice of intuition. It is a voice that is kind, that allows you to take a break, book the trip, or schedule your massage. This voice of intuition, of knowing, or your higher guidance and direction can be noticed by its characteristics of being calm, kind, loving, supportive, reassuring and gentle. Essentially, when you hear this voice you will feel good or, at least, better. You can trust this voice to guide you.

When your gremlin voice shows up, notice how it makes you feel. The hallmark of the gremlin versus intuition is that the gremlin makes you feel bad. There is good news though. You can talk to it. For instance, you can say, "I see you're showing up again but this isn't helpful to me right now. Instead, I'm going to listen to this deeper voice within—the kinder one." Or, "I hear what you're saying, but...." Start to find ways to reframe and become less attached to that gremlin voice. It can be helpful to name it, so you can recognize it is part of you, but not all of you. It's separate from the Truth of who you are.

With this awareness, I can now look upon the voice and appreciate that it was trying to protect me when I was younger and believed I didn't fit in. But the truth now is that I'm okay. I've got this. I can appreciate that it helped me be so driven to accomplish all I have, and at the same time ask for it to be a little bit quieter so I can enjoy who I am. It no longer needs to rob me of my joy in a relentless pursuit of impossible perfection.

If this feels weird, it's okay. It did for me at first too, yet in learning how to notice, accept, and gently reassign the role of my gremlin voice, I have seen a huge improvement in my mental state of wellbeing.

Confidence isn't something you have to wait to get. You can regain it—or start building it—today by better understanding your value(s) and through learning a new way to interact with the voice inside your head. Head over to the workbook to get started.

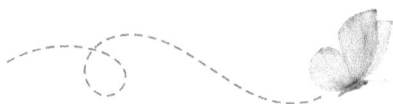

Chapter Ten

Self-care to Sustain

The old idea of feeling guilty for taking care of ourselves has to die. Today. For centuries, women have suffered at the hands of the belief that, "I must put others' needs before and above mine." If everyone else is comfortable, cared for, and resting, then—and only then—may I have time for myself. We don't give ourselves permission because we are last on the list. We have put others before ourselves, and then wonder why we feel exhausted, resentful, and worn down.

Maybe you've recognized a need for balance and made steps towards incorporating your self-care rituals while also making sure the important people in your life are cared for. You're on the right track. I'm going to request, though, that you take this a step further. Our self-care is no longer a luxury. It's not something we do just when we have time, after the cups of others have been filled, or as a fleeting goal.

Self-care is critical for our evolution as women. Leaning on the accolades of acknowledgment from others to give us the "boost" we needed should no longer be relied on to sustain us. We cannot fill other cups before ours. It's not sustainable, and it won't last—at least, not without significant health and happiness consequences.

As we evolve into the women we desire to be, we need to fill our cups daily, and on an ongoing basis. When we feel whole, balanced, and energized, then we can give of ourselves to others. This is the new paradigm of self-care and it is anything but selfish. It's a requirement for our flourishing, and for those around us.

We must put our oxygen mask on first.

Next time you find yourself feeling down, or stuck in a spiral of negative emotions, remember that this is your conditioned, catabolic, primitive mind that once protected you from experiencing the worst-case scenario. Then use one of these ways to move forward. They're free, they're fast—in case you're short on time and cash—and are beautiful ways to care for yourself physically, mentally, and emotionally.

FUTURE-SELF JOURNAL

Future-self journaling is a practice I use daily; it allows me to create, on paper, the experiences and feelings I want to have in my most ideal life. The practice is to envision your dreamiest life, down to the detail of how you interact with your spouse and kids, how meaningful your friendships are, how you show up at work, and all the abundance you get to enjoy. You write as though you are already living your dream.

Envision how your future self feels about herself and her life. Be sure to write about it in the present tense. This practice, although it may sound strange, collapses the quantum field of possibility and begins to create the life and reality you want. For me, this can sound like,

Work is easy and fun for me. My relationships are flourishing. I feel deeply connected to those I most love, and money flows to me with ease. I feel great about all I've accomplished, about who I am, and I'm able to show up, unapologetically, as my whole Self. I trust my kind heart and compassionate approach to always guide me in relationships. I'm loved and I am being guided. My needs are taken care of, always.

And other times, it's less fluffy, sounding something like,

This life is so f*cking amazing! I love my body, my friends, my amazing home, and my ability to travel every single

month to a beautiful new place. Life is full of cool people, great clothes, and amazing wine. I love that we're building our dream home in the mountains, and it's all easy and fun.

If you need help getting into a creative mindset before future-self journaling, download and listen to this free meditation that is guided by my dear friend and Transformation Coach, Betsy Weiner.

kindlcoaching.com/
aob-resource

RANT FOR RELIEF

For the times when my negative talk can't be wiped away with future-self journaling, I go to another favorite—a rant. Before you call me crazy or get confused, let me explain. We often avoid difficult feelings by escaping them in order to immediately feel better. What doesn't get resolved though, are the lingering-beneath-the-surface, shitty feelings that keep coming up. When I have these lingering-beneath-the-surface, shitty days, or moments, no amount of gratitude journaling or future-self journaling is going to get me there. On these days, I know it's time to rant. Instead of bottling them up, I let them come pouring out!

This process is about acknowledging and accepting what is, even if you hate to admit it. For me, it might sound like,

I hate my work. My family is impossible to be around. My kids are a pain in the ass. My life sucks. I feel fat and ugly. I'm a loner. I look old, and suck at what I do. No one values my work.

As you can see, it's not pretty, and it's not fun, but it is honest.

What happens when we stop avoiding difficult feelings and face them head on is a deep acceptance of what is. It is in this powerful acceptance and letting it all out that the energy of our deep pain moves through us, and no longer has a hold on us. If we avoid it at all costs, it builds in strength and we don't get to learn the resilience and strength we have within by facing and successfully moving through difficult and fearful times.

If you're not much of a writer, try a voice-recorded rant. Whether writing or speaking the harshest of words that are trapped within and need to come out, you are learning to release and accept what is instead of pretending it isn't there, covering it up with avoidance, immersing yourself in work, or toxic positivity—saying you're "great" when you're not. By releasing your darkest feelings onto the page, you release it from your life. You will feel lighter on the other side of it. Yes, you may have to come back to this practice many times, but you'll see that with each honest declaration of how much you suck, you will, paradoxically, feel better. It's a simple but powerful form of self-care.

COLD SHOWER

Another quick and easy form of self-care you can integrate into your day is taking a cold shower. Before you start shivering at the idea of even considering this, let me explain.

Taking a cold shower, even for just a few minutes has massive benefits including boosting your energy and metabolism and helping to detoxify your body. One less-often considered benefit is the ability to begin clearing your mind. We often default to reactivity in our lives. Someone says something hurtful, we feel ashamed. Someone cuts us off in traffic, we get angry. Our kids talk back, we get pissed.

A cold shower helps us practice the art of detaching from an immediate reaction to a more thoughtful response. It's like taking a breath, or a pause, from the conditioned response to consider how we want to be. The cold shower is a perfect training ground to move from the, "Shit this is cold, this sucks, this sucks. I'm freezing!" reaction to focusing our attention onto something else. Our minds are powerful and can focus on whatever we choose. Why not choose better-feeling thoughts than, "This sucks" in the shower and in life?

During my two-minute daily cold shower, I divert my attention to brushing my teeth. I start with a warm shower while I shampoo and condition my hair and wash my face. Then I turn the shower as cold as it can go and begin brushing my teeth while counting. Every thirty seconds, I switch "sides" of my body under the cold water, as well as the area of my mouth I'm brushing.

For example, I'll start out with the cold water on the front of my body, neck down, while brushing the top row, outside part of my teeth. Counting one-to-thirty. When I get to thirty, I rotate to the left side of my body, now cleaning the inside of my top row of teeth, and the process continues for approximately two minutes. On more ambitious days, I may wash up, then rinse my body and hair in the cold shower for some added shine. I then turn the water back to warm and finish my comfortable shower. I've learned to breathe through my nose and embrace the cold.

Thinking about things other than how uncomfortable that moment is an incredible way to train your brain. It's a daily practice that is teaching me I can change my thoughts anytime throughout the day and in life.

This simple practice is a powerful way to begin to shift your mind from focusing on the pain, to move toward acceptance. You can find peace in discomfort and bring yourself back to a place of control. It's a practice that teaches you that your reaction to what happens in your external environment is up to you. You can choose to freak out, say you can't do it, or hate every minute of your two-minute cool down. Or you can choose to breathe, surrender, find peace, and create the ability to think about something else. Your mind doesn't have to become all-consumed with the frigid water washing over you.

And don't forget the added benefit of the daily metabolism and energy boost you will get.

Interestingly, by integrating these few simple practices into my life, my "bounce-back" rate has improved.

I still get drained from giving more of myself to my family and work than what was in my cup to give. I know when I'm here because I feel down, believe that life sucks, or that the cards are stacked against me. In these moments, instead of remaining a victim to life's curve balls, or being unaware of overextending myself, I can pick one of these guilt-free forms of self-care to get me back to baseline. It's not always immediate, but it helps.

It has also taught me that my emotions, no matter how extreme, how amazing, or how difficult, come and go. None of them are permanent. None of them define me. And none of them define you. You are a beautiful, complex, passionate woman, and as you ride the waves of life, you will get to experience the highest of highs and the lowest of lows.

Ultimately, when you prioritize yourself and your energy, you are refueled and can continue to show up for others. This is one of the most selfless things you can do. It's a beautiful act of care for not only you, but for everyone you deeply care about.

Remember that when the dark clouds come, you can pick one of these methods to experiment with what works best for you. Pain is inevitable, but the ongoing suffering is optional. You get to choose how you move yourself up and out of the darkest days of your life. Having these tools at your disposal, whenever you need them, is a beautiful way to put yourself first when you need it most.

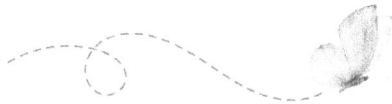

Chapter Eleven

Age with Grace

B efore you read this chapter, download this meditation guided by Betsy Weiner. It will guide you to the
highest vision for yourself, which will help you set your
intention for how to Age with Grace in the highest way
for yourself.

kindlcoaching.com/
aob-resource

Part of Aging with Grace is aging with a feeling of loving acceptance toward yourself and your body, regardless of the changes you are experiencing. After completing this meditation, focus on the highest vision for yourself. This is the vision of the woman that you desire to be and all that you get to experience leading the life you want to lead. It's similar to taking the future-self journaling practice from the last chapter to the next level. With practice, you can start to create this as a reality in your life today.

Aging with Grace requires an ongoing practice of choosing loving, supportive, nurturing thoughts over the fearful gremlin voice inside you. As a reminder, this is as simple as noticing when you are feeling bad, down, or any other undesired emotion. When you recognize it, you can decide that it's not the truth of who you are, at least not fully. You can then choose a more calming, supportive thought. This ongoing choice of picking the loving voice or the loving decision over the fearful one is a practice which will allow you to Age with Grace.

The first step is learning how to integrate instead of avoiding pain in your life. It may sound counterintuitive, but I've learned firsthand that, when practiced, I can take back control of my life and reduce my reactivity to old triggers.

INTEGRATE PAIN

There's a way of integrating painful experiences that is different from the typical avoidance approach we default to in our lives. When we are able to integrate past painful experiences that have an emotional hold on us, we release their grip, much like we learned to release the grip of the controlling gremlin voice.

Take a moment to recall a painful experience of your past. Instead of the easier, habitual route of avoiding it, or pretending it doesn't exist, I want you to focus on it, and then use one of the two techniques below to integrate it into your life with the goal of letting it go, slowly, over time.

The first practice is one I learned from Michael Singer in his book, *The Untethered Soul* (2013):

With your painful experience identified clearly in your mind, recognize where you notice that pain in your body. Is it in your shoulder, your throat, your stomach? Wherever it is, envision it as though it's a thorn in your skin. The more you resist it by tightening your muscles around it or recounting the pain in your mind, the deeper the thorn drives into your skin. It stays. What you resist, persists. Find a safe and comfortable place to feel this emotion, this thorn, and begin to release the tension it has on you, literally and figuratively.

I get into the bath or find a comfortable spot on the floor to allow myself to breathe and relax into the tense emotion in my body. First, I bring the tough feeling to the forefront of my mind. Then I notice where I feel the most tension or restriction and envision the thorn right there. In the safety of my home, I allow anything and everything around that tension to come up and out. This often involves crying, recalling how hurt, saddened, and alone I feel. Yet, I continue to breathe and continue to relax into it and allow all feelings to come up. Sometimes I feel rageful, hateful, and frustrated. Other times, I need to yell, to say the things that I didn't have the courage to say before, as a way to release. It's intense and it can feel uncomfortable. I continue breathing, relaxing, and allowing. After a few minutes, the most pressing feelings have released, and I feel a bit lighter, a bit more free.

That's all it takes, a few minutes of time for you to feel your emotions. It is a powerful way to release the tension that has been there but has been showing up in less predictable ways. By facing your discomfort here, on your terms, on your timeline, and in your chosen safe location, you get to take control of the pain through mindful integration instead of letting it control you.

The second practice is one I learned from Gabrielle Bernstein in her book, *The Universe Has Your Back* (2016). It involves much of the same preparation.

Recognize and bring the painful experience, along with all the overwhelming emotions, to the forefront of your mind. Then, envision yourself walking into the shallows of the ocean, standing in the water of the emotion. As you

stand there, with each inhale, see waves of overwhelming
   fear, emotion, and uncertainty coming toward you. As it
approaches, allow yourself to feel the gravity and fullness
of that emotion, and then either jump over or dive through
the wave, exhaling and standing on the other side. Envision
the next wave of emotion flowing toward you on the inhale,
move through it on your exhale, and continue the process,
   allowing the waves to wash by you.

What I have noticed through this practice is that the wave intensity lessens with each subsequent wave, validating that when we accept and integrate our waves of pain, instead of fearfully standing on the shore and pretending they aren't there, they lessen their hold on us.

CHOOSE YOUR AGE

An important key to Aging with Grace is reframing how you see yourself through the inevitable process of change. There are other ways you can embody the fullness of who you are as a woman, regardless of your age. To do that, I'd like to introduce you to four different ways in which you can define your age. Then you can see which one you've been identifying with, perhaps shamefully or with resistance. These include your chronological, biological, emotional, and spiritual ages.

Your chronological age is how many years you've been alive. But certainly, this has its limitations. Some people only live for a short while, while others live well into their 100s. Putting a simple number to what may seem like a linear timeline is extremely limiting. It gives no perspective on your vitality, your good years ahead, or all the experience you've gained so far. It's just a number. It tells nothing of how much time is left. You could be eighty and living your best years yet, or never make it to that number. So while it is helpful as a frame of reference, it does not encompass the fullness of your life. And it's a metric that you have zero control over. It's just a number.

Your biological age is a representation of your physical health and vitality. It can serve as an indication of your vibrant time left relative to the choices you are making in your life. Bottom line, this number is in your control. There are countless ways to reduce your biological age, increase your longevity, and improve your health for whatever time you do have. To describe this in greater detail, I'd like to share a story of two acquaintances.

A surfing buddy of mine loathed the idea of aging. She complained about it almost anytime the topic of birthdays or fun activities came up. When we went surfing, she suggested she better do it now, before she's too old to get up on the board. When we celebrated a friend's birthday, she mentioned how she wasn't looking forward to her next birthday because it just meant she was getting older.

Truth be told, she looked and acted old. She was holding onto a belief of her limited capacity and, therefore, slumped her shoulders, didn't try new activities she was fully capable of and was forever trying the latest anti-aging thing to look and feel younger. She acted and looked old. When I once asked her age, I was surprised to learn she was just thirty-six at the time. If I had to guess, I would have thought she was in her fifties. Her biological age, based on her limiting beliefs about her age-related restrictions, was causing her to age faster than necessary.

Conversely, a grandfather to one of our son's friends on his soccer team is ninety-one years old. He walks eight miles per day, shows up to every soccer game with his wife, and still lives independently. He's full of energy, full of life. His biological age seems much less than a typical ninety-one-year-old. He's got lots of living left to do, and both his mindset and activity levels only improve these numbers. His biological age is quite lower than his chronological age, and he has made many life choices to support this.

Another way to identify age is emotional. It's how you act. Are you someone who sits deep in contemplation, making sense of things like the meaning of life? Do you tend to take things seriously, as I often do? These can be indicators of an older emotional age, a seriousness, and an adult-like responsibility of helping, serving, and supporting others.

Or, are you a carefree kid emotionally? Do you live in the moment, laugh and play, and prioritize fun over completing tasks? Do you skip with your kids, or take time away from work to jump with them on the trampoline? So often, we live with so much heaviness and responsibility in our lives that dampen our innate desire to be free and fully enjoy the ride of life. Perhaps it's time to consider the things that weigh you down, keep you serious and adult-like, and find more fun in your day as a way to feel emotionally younger.

And finally, spiritual age is a representation of the everlasting, infinite soul within you. Based on spiritual beliefs, this may be your ever-lasting life, your higher Self, your spirit that lives on. While your body may perish, your consciousness and awareness live on. Or perhaps you don't believe in something greater than you, but can acknowledge since energy cannot be created or destroyed—and you are an energetic being—that when you die, your energy will shift forms. Part of you will live on, even if it changes form over time.

This is your spiritual Self, your spiritual age, and it is infinite.

Are you an "old soul" like our son who, despite being a teenager, says the most profound things, as though he has been around before? Do you have moments of déjà vu, where you know you have experienced something before, even though it could not have possibly occurred in this lifetime?

You are not defined by the narrow limits of a calendar-defined age, but have several options available to you in how you perceive yourself, and even represent your age emotionally, biologically, and spiritually.

HEALTH

Some believe declining health is an inevitable part of aging. While it may be true that our bodies will eventually stop functioning in their current capacity, you have a lot more influence on your health than you may realize. I invite you to begin noticing your language on health. Remember, what we focus on is what we attract more of into our lives. So, if you're complaining about your back pain or a new knee injury, your focus will go there. Unfortunately, you will experience more of it. Yes, you will inevitably have changes to your health, pain levels, and diagnoses as you age, but instead of battling the negative, focus on what you want instead.

Terms like "battling cancer," "controlling Crohn's flare ups," "fighting pain," or even "relieving pain," focus on the negative, the illness, the disease, and what is undesirable.

Instead, change your language to what you want to attract more of. Focus on the good stuff in your life. This is how the Law of Resonance, sometimes called the Law of Attraction, works. So, instead of saying, "I'm battling my cancer," or "I'm cancer-free," choose something that feels true to you but more empowering. Perhaps this could sound like, "I'm embodying health," "My body heals itself," or "I have the support I need to be healthy and strong."

When you focus on your language, you begin to change and shape the narrative, and the truth is that our bodies are self-healing when they have the right support. Part of the support is the words you are using when you talk about health.

A family friend was recently diagnosed with brain cancer and is in the hospital for chemotherapy every other week, missing huge milestones like his daughter's graduation and dropping her off at college. However, when asked how he's doing, he is more radiant and appreciative than ever. He is truly, deeply grateful for the outpouring of love and support he has received. He appreciates getting to see a new, more loving side to friends. He loves his daughters more than ever. He loves his wife more than ever. He, of course, would never wish cancer on anyone, yet wishes everyone could experience the awakening that he has. And while none of us can predict the future, my belief is that his focus on all the beauty and blessings that surround him will only help his prognosis.

"Focus on what you love to create more of it" is a beautiful and inspiring motto to live by.

It's crucial that whatever you are saying, you must truly believe it, or it won't work. So, no matter how small the shift toward the positive, make one that you believe is possible. If you repeat it in conversation with others, or anytime the topic of your health comes up, you will begin to witness the power of your positive thoughts. Your healing language will work its magic in your life.

To dig deeper, notice where you feel symptoms in your body, then breathe into and feel that part of your body, and ask yourself what that pain/part would say if it could speak. What does it have to tell you? Then listen. Whatever you first hear, think, or notice is what it's saying.

Listen to it, believe it, and then take the actions necessary to support what comes up. For example, when I tune in and ask why I have ongoing shoulder tension, then listen, what I hear is, "You push too much. You make life harder than it needs to be. You judge too much of what is happening and where you are in life, and it's not meant to be this hard. Whenever you are tense in your shoulders, remember you are pushing. Life doesn't have to be this way. It can be easier, more fun."

Based on this knowledge, I now notice my shoulder tension, and recognize that instead of pushing through toward a writing deadline or continuing to pick up the house, something needs to shift. I need to shift. So, I'll close my laptop and go have fun, take a walk, snuggle my dogs, or listen to music to change the vibe in my body and in my life. This practice might sound weird, but it works. Give it a try and see what comes up for you.

It's a practice, but instead of focusing on aging or your energy being lower, much like you're learning to do with your health, you can shift your focus onto all that is good.

What are you grateful for, or appreciative of? What do you have that's going well for you? What are the parts of you that you love, genuinely?

When you shift your focus from what is undesired to what is desired, it might feel disingenuous at first. But keep at it and attract more of what you do want, instead of what you don't into your life.

An example of this is my hyperfocus on the number on the scale. By constantly focusing on, and thinking about, my weight, I am creating more weight. In these times, the scale creeps up. Conversely, when I focus on how good I feel, how energized I am, or the parts of my body that I like, I notice I not only feel better but the scale drops as well. The power of our minds is immense, and when we choose more loving, positive thoughts toward what we want in our lives and actually believe it's possible, the magic is incredible.

Focus on whatever it is that you want more of, instead of the thing you do not.

There are many ways to age beautifully and gracefully, and so much of it is in your perception, thoughts, and language around this inevitable shift. You have the power to choose, moment to moment, how you think and speak. It's not a switch you flip to suddenly feel great about getting older, but with practice, you will feel more empowered in your life—and more loving toward yourself.

Remember, Baby, you're worth it !!

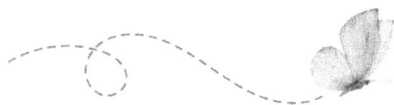

Chapter Twelve

Becoming Timeless

There is a timeless quality to beauty. It is a presence, an inner radiance. The beauty industry attempts to capture this by showcasing a youthful, radiant model with flawless, blurred, yet lit-from-within skin, or the golden tones and wardrobe of a goddess-like woman. And while it may seem elusive to you beyond the highlighter and blurring/perfecting powder, the truth is that you can create this timelessness in your life, regardless of age, through practices of presence, purpose, and becoming more playful.

PRESENCE

To embody this timeless quality, you can first and foremost become more present in your life. When we think about time ticking on, the limited amount of time we have, or are stuck in our heads in the past or future, we certainly aren't here, in this moment. Unknowingly, we are accelerating time because we are moving through life without the attention and appreciation of the beauty right in front of us.

Through practice, you too can learn to become more present in your life, in a way that's deeply powerful. When you move out of your thinking mind and, instead, observe without judgment or labels, you can create a sense of time slowing down. Read that sentence again, slowly, and breathe deeply as you do.

Time becomes non-existent when you are truly, fully here in the present. Anything that exists outside what is right here in front of us is only a mental construct in our mind. The past only exists in what is re-lived in our mind's memories—through our rehashing of or recollection of a prior event.

Similarly, the future also only exists in our minds. When deep in thought of what might be or considering how we "should" be preparing for the meeting, these thoughts feel so real, such a big part of who we are. Yet the truth is that there's no part of us that will ever be able to live in the past or the future. Any amount of time we spend other than in this moment—right here—is taking us away from our timeless, ethereal quality. It's taking us away from our present experience. And it's taking our energy away as it's diverted toward things that are not in front of us.

While this idea of presence sounds good, it can be difficult to learn how to integrate it into your life in a meaningful way. After reading this chapter, head to the workbook to notice the thoughts that are rooted in the past, in the here and now, and in the future. Generally speaking, when we are thinking about the past or the future, there's a negative or fearful thought around it which, therefore, reduces our energy.

Part of becoming timeless is recognizing that when you're fully in the present moment, time stops, your physical body is here and, because your higher Self is not being distracted by the egoic, primitive mind or other controlling thoughts, you become in alignment. When you're in alignment, your energy shines brighter and your radiance is more visible. You resonate at a higher, more anabolic, energy level. Not only does this create more presence and timelessness, but it also attracts more good things to you.

Meaning, you'll start to see more of the beauty in and around your life as you practice this spiritual journey of becoming more present in your own life.

BE ON PURPOSE

The second part of becoming timeless is identifying and living out your purpose to any degree possible—even if it's as a hobby in your spare time. So many of us go through life with a misguided version of what it means to be on purpose. It all centers around accomplishing, doing, and meeting all of the expectations that were placed upon us from an early age.

But when we go inward, we begin to understand our inherent worth in who we are without all the "doing." By going deeper into our authentic Self and living into our purpose, we start to see that the human we are being is enough. And when we're living a life built around our meaning, then the pushiness, heaviness, and diffi- culty of living a life out of alignment starts to become aligned. It starts to feel easier. Instead of pushing, and living with constant shoulder tension, you start to feel like you're being pulled toward something that is truly, deeply meaningful to you.

Purpose is found at the intersection of what you most value, what you enjoy doing, and what you're good at. Be sure to head to the workbook to revisit your values, then make a list of the things you really love doing that naturally raise your energy and vibe. Then consider all that you're good at.

Don't hold back. Recall all you have accomplished that you are naturally gifted at, that perhaps comes easy, or that others have recognized you for. This task isn't easy, and takes time, yet is well worth the effort. There's no need to overthink this, as we can have multiple different purposes throughout life and at any given time. When you live out your purpose, you become more timeless because time can stand still, be enjoyable, and give you energy, creating more fullness in your life.

BE A KID

Finally, we are going to revisit the definitions of age—to become more timeless, and have fun in the process. Sure, the limiting chronological age that you used to get so worked up about will tick on no matter what. Remember, it's only a number, and it's so limited in its capacity to define the truth of who you are as a woman.

A bigger part of being timeless is being free to have fun, play, run around, and be a kid, doing the things that make you happy, free, joyful, and connected with those you most love. Remember how, as a child, before all the conditioning that you went through, you were pure love? You were free; you were curious; you were joyful. You were quite young emotionally, yet were living close to your spirituality, closer to the Truth of You—the Spiritual You. When you do that, you create undeniable high-vibe energy. You will be present in what you're doing because you're having fun with it and there's no capacity for more limiting and negative thoughts to come in. You become timeless in the presence of your emotional youth.

For me, this looks like skipping down the street with my kids, or sometimes by myself, not caring what my neighbors think, or saying "yes" when my son asks me to head down the waterslide or play soccer. These are fun choices that build connection and get me out of my serious, adult-like, "doing" mind. They're usually filled with shared laughter and stories.

You can become timeless in your biological age, but I want to caution that if you become overly focused on biohacking your age down, on decreasing that number because you are inherently feeling old, then it's not going to be as powerful.

Redefining how you view your body, and how you want to listen to, nourish, support, and trust it can do wonders. It is exhausting to feel like your body can't be trusted, like you have to fight against it with the foods you put in your mouth, reach for the latest supplement, or control the weight on the scale.

When you love and trust your body for the vessel and vehicle that it is, for all it allows you to do and experience, your biological age is naturally going to decrease without the effort and controlling habit we fall into. As a child, you certainly weren't preoccupied with the calorie count of the snack you reached for. You ate when you were hungry, then ran back outside to play. You were in flow, trusting yourself and your body. You can come back to this freedom and trust any time.

As we talked about before, there's a part of you that lives on forever. Your spiritual age is infinite—a part of you that's everlasting. When you think about being timeless, the truth is: that is who you already are. Stacy Hartmann teaches in her book *Metaconscious Entrepreneur*, "You can be 100 percent spiritual and 100 percent human at the same time" (Hartmann 2021).

While your humanness has a chronological age, your spirituality does not. It lives on. It is timeless. It already is these things without even having to be, do, or strive to become anything different. This alternate way of viewing yourself is here to help you recognize there is an ethereal, beautiful, timeless quality to you that you get to focus on and enjoy—or completely disregard—in your life. That choice is yours.

Because I'm on this journey with you, I want to share a story that caught me by surprise. I've been doing the same work that I talk about in this book, and it's been a wild ride, but I'm here to reassure you this is all possible.

We were recently invited to a progressive boat dinner where we traveled from house to house via boat. It was super fun, a beautiful day, and the weather was gorgeous outside, as we returned to our starting home after picnic-style dinners at each of the three host houses. We were on the dock, getting the boats unloaded and picked up, when out of the blue, one of our acquaintances said, "You know, Casie, you just have this aura about you. You've got this light and this brightness about you and above you."

As he motioned to the space above my head, he said, "I just wanted to say, it's really nice." It seemed to come out of nowhere, and yet, it hit so deeply at my core because I'd been paid such a beautiful compliment when I least expected it. Another guy chimed in from the boat he was organizing to say, "Yeah Casie, you do! You've got a great aura!" Laughing and smiling at the same time, I said, "Thank you!" These guys are big, masculine dudes. Great husbands and fathers, but certainly not the type of guys I would have ever expected to notice someone's aura! Of all of the compliments I could have been paid, it wasn't, "You've got a great smile," "You're fun to be around," or, "We love you guys." It was none of that. It was about my aura, my presence coming from a spiritual light. I was surprised at how noticeable this light had become even to people not used to looking for something like this. It was a compliment that, I believe, could have only been seen by others due to the work I had been doing on myself.

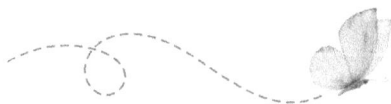

Chapter Thirteen

Fulfillment and Happiness

U nderstanding your purpose raises your level of fulfillment. Knowing your purpose and what brings
you joy can create new opportunities to appreciate
where you are in life. For example, if you value connection, you may choose to get together once per month
with your closest girlfriends. If you love teaching and
dancing, you may volunteer at a dance studio. Maybe
you get out your old painting supplies, or sign up for
a hip-hop class, learn to garden, or whatever it is that
lights you up. It doesn't need to be a big shift, like
quitting your job to pursue your passion, or considering
a more fulfilling partnership.

Fulfillment isn't a destination you reach. Life is dy-
namic and so is fulfillment. It is a subtle and intention-

al shift toward creating more contentment in your life. Much like the pursuit of happiness, you don't fully arrive at a blissful, happy state and then stay there. Part of what creates our ability to feel fulfilled is to also have fully experienced the lows. It's the relative shift that offers the ability to truly feel the highs. In other words, without the lows we wouldn't notice, and therefore appreciate, the highs. Yet beyond just embracing the lows, there is much within your control that can help move you in this direction.

As you become more fulfilled through minor shifts in how you're spending your time, your happiness levels will naturally follow suit. But, if you're ready to create more "Happier-ness," here's how to do it.

BECOMING HAPPIER

Notice how you think about your pursuit of happiness. If you're constantly talking about, or thinking about, how you will be happy when _____ happens to or for you, then you are sending out waves to the universe that you are not currently happy. You are essentially stating that you aren't happy now and need something in your external environment to change to become happy. You are giving all your power away. You are approaching it from a place of lack. And unfortunately, you will create more of what you focus on. More things to be unhappy about. It's counterintuitive, but it's a universal law and one you can shift, starting today, to create more happiness in your life.

A former colleague of mine has a default tendency toward unhappiness. She often feels stressed about her weight, that she's drinking too much, frustrated with her husband for his travel schedule, and angry at her leadership team for their chosen direction. I remember her sharing details of her childhood where she noticed the problems in herself and others, with high degrees of judgment.

This is one of the ways she learned to keep herself safe and protected. If she could stay ahead of her mother's criticism, by first judging herself and then changing everything possible about who she was to meet some false, external standard set by her, then she would be "safe" and "okay." The problem is that this perspective is no longer serving her. Instead, she is living a life of less-than, of hyper-focus on the things she doesn't like about herself, her life, her job, and her marriage.

This focus is keeping her in a state of lack, of less than, of needing to change in order to be okay. But will it ever come? I believe it will. The moment she recognizes that "efforting"—or pushing to be and do more—and judging every step of the way is actually holding her back from her true Self, she can unlock the next level. By creating a simple shift in perspective and starting to focus on the good in her life, the world around her will shift too.

Suddenly, she will be able to see more of the beauty in who she already is. The beauty in her job, her marriage, her life. She can enjoy the ride of her life by focusing on all that is good. Sure, she has moments of bliss; when she gets recognized at work, goes for a morning run, or is planning her next vacation. But she quickly moves back to her default state of unhappiness. It's difficult to watch someone I care about in her struggle, while knowing I can help her shift and change perspective. Yet I have learned to accept that everyone comes to these realizations in their own time and in their own ways. She knows I'm here when she's ready, and that's all that matters.

The other default state you can choose is one of hap-piness. It's not about being happy all the time—that's not life. Life will continue to throw curve balls, cause pain, and struggle. But a baseline state of happiness builds resilience, perspective and, dare I say, even appreciation for what happens in life, because it can be seen through a lens of learning, growth, and momentary impact. Prac-ticing feeling good brings your default state to one of happiness; a state that with a simple movement you can come back to easily.

A client of mine embodies this beautifully. She has had incredible setbacks in her life, including a long journey through infertility and multiple miscarriages. She has lost loved ones, gone through divorce, taken a demotion at work and, like all of us, struggles with aging. Yet despite these life experiences, she remains hopeful, optimistic, and forward-moving in her life. She views each setback as just that—a momentary distraction from her life before she comes back to baseline. She has learned through our work together that even the emotional hold of the most tragic of experiences can be reframed and released to achieve even greater levels of happiness.

It's a beautiful journey, a beautiful unfolding to witness, and inspiring to be around.

What we often don't realize is that this level of happiness is a choice we get to make, every day and in every situation. It's as simple as this: notice your default, and then make a choice to shift your focus from one of lack to appreciation for what is. See the good in yourself and others. Trust that better days are ahead instead of waiting for the other shoe to drop. It might sound overly simplistic, yet with consistent practice in redirecting your thoughts from the negative to a positive, believable aspect of whatever person or situation you are faced with, you will, over time, see your default state begin to shift from unhappy to happy.

Head over to the workbook to reflect upon your default state. Don't worry if it's more unhappy than you'd like to admit. There is much you can do to shift this in your pursuit of happier-ness. As you move toward greater levels of happiness in your life, you'll become more resilient, better able to see learning in even the most difficult of situations, and more trusting of others and of your life's unfolding. And the best part is that your whole journey of becoming will be more enjoyable.

LOVE IS ALL YOU NEED

Beyond the guise of being happier, I believe The Beatles were spot on when they sang, *All You Need Is Love*. Beneath the desire to be happier is, ultimately, the desire to be loved. Let me explain. Say you are awaiting your promotion, new car, more money, better relationship, better body, more radiant skin, or the warmth of summer to be happy. Really, under all of that, you are looking for more acceptance and connection with others, and beyond that, love.

With this recognition, we can start to look at the things that we expect, or want, to change in our lives in order to be happy; to understand what feeling that new role, new car, fitter body, or smoother skin will create for us. In this process, we will recognize that all the things you have been dependent on for your happiness are really just a means to an end.

They are there to create certain desired feelings, including love and acceptance, through the having or achieving of that thing. Yet the "thing" was never an end in and of itself. It was only a goal to get you closer to feelings of fullness, completeness, and acceptance of who you are. With this knowledge, you can find alternate ways to create these feelings in your life. Or, to recognize many of them are already here, you simply need to ac-knowledge and enjoy them. You have control over your feelings. Therefore, in an adjustment of your thoughts and feelings, through practices like meditation, gratitude journaling, future-self journaling, or ranting can allow you to release the feelings that you don't like, in favor of those that feel better.

FIVE KEYS

I learned through my coaching education at iPEC that there are five basic keys to happiness.

Know you can weather your moods.

Choose balance without judgment.

Develop support systems.

Challenge yourself to grow.

Define yourself and express your gifts.

Let's break them down, shall we?

Know You Can Weather Your Moods

Life is a roller-coaster of ups and downs and all-arounds. Yet, how many times have you let yourself spiral?

On a bad day, when something goes wrong, you start spiraling into, "Why did I say that?" "I should have thought more before I spoke," "I'm such an idiot," "I'll probably get passed up for the next opportunity," "Same old same old," "My boss favors him anyway," "Ugh—I hate my job," "The house is a mess," "I've got so much to do," "I'm totally overwhelmed," "My husband never helps," "So much has to change," "Everything has to change." What started with a simple mistake in a meeting spiraled into an entire dislike for your life. If you're like me, this spiral can happen quickly and be hard to catch, until you're sulking in a sea of self-pity, frustration, and helplessness.

Yet, when I recognize that we all have good and bad days and times on the roller-coaster of life, I can let the original thought be, or maybe spiral a little but without all the ongoing judgment that keeps me there. I can acknowledge that maybe I should have thought more before I chimed in at the meeting—but who cares? Everyone makes mistakes. It's not a big deal and I doubt anyone else is still thinking about it. This perspective shift does two things. First, it helps me remember that life is a series of ups and downs, and I'll be up again, on fire, having a great day. And second, that I don't have to stay in the down. Even that is a choice.

So, the biggest key to knowing you can weather your moods is remembering that the ups are great, the downs are normal, and it's all okay. You're okay. You don't have to judge yourself for the down time. You can, instead, accept it and know the upswing will follow suit. Ironically, the faster you integrate and accept the "bad," the faster you bounceback. The pain is inevitable, but the suffering of it is optional, and it's all related to how much you judge yourself in the "downs."

Choose Balance Without Judgment

How often do you feel guilty for your non-doing, for your relaxation, for your "slacking"?

I used to judge these things a lot, feeling guilty for almost anything I'd do for "me" during working hours; I had to be on all the time, giving 110%. I judged myself if I got sick. I felt guilty if I needed to duck out early to pick up my kids. I worried my boss would call when I was getting my nails done at 4:55pm. I didn't allow myself to relax, take a break, or have balance, because I felt guilty when I did, and certainly didn't enjoy my "down time."

This perspective left me stuck, multitasking my life away, but not in a fun or fluid way.

It was a frantic, fearful energy of not-enoughness, and it caused me to spill my coffee on the way out the door, trip over my dog, and snap at the kids. It's the energy that made my heart race and my anxiety soar. I occasionally chose "balance," but always with self-judgment. I've since learned that balance is normal, necessary, and required to self-sustain. It's a beautiful practice when I can support myself, fully enjoy my "me time," and trust that I'll return to life more energized and refreshed in a way that benefits everyone.

I've released the expectation that I can, and should, do it all in favor of asking for help without shame. I've exchanged the idea of inattentive multitasking for fuller presence, to whatever or whomever is right in front of me. I've replaced my self-judgment with self-love, reminding myself it's not only okay to love and care for myself but it is also necessary, honorable, and setting a great example.

I now get to enjoy my massages, recognize that I have off days where I need to rest and recover, and love the opportunity to binge-watch *Emily in Paris* as part of my recharge. I have a choice in my balance and rest, and I certainly don't have to judge it. You, too, can release your self-judgment in favor of more loving and supportive thoughts in your pursuit of happier-ness.

Develop Support Systems

Since 1938, The Harvard Study on Adult Development (Waldinger, ongoing study), has been investigating what makes people flourish. As the longest in-depth study on adult life, it has concluded that close relationships are the most important factor in happiness and well-being. So, who are your go-to homies that you can literally say and share anything with? The people who stand by your side, whether you're feeling on-top-of-the-world and excited to celebrate your latest win, or in the lowest of lows, feeling afraid, uncertain, and vulnerable. Who can you cry your eyes out to, knowing that they will hold space for you, no matter what?

These are the people beyond the fun, social, "cheers"-type friends, who are there when you are doing well, ready to listen to the latest band or go out for a cocktail. These are the friends who have your back, no matter what. They accept you as the whole of you. Another important consideration for developing your support system is to understand who in your life gains or drains your energy. Knowing how important high vibe energy is for feeling your best, most beautiful, badass self as you age, you want to surround yourself with other high-energy people. Head over to the workbook to identify those people in your life that you most deeply connect with.

Challenge Yourself To Grow

This might sound morbid, but if we don't grow, we die. A key to being happy is to challenge yourself to grow, always. Part of what this learning mindset embodies is a notion of curiosity instead of judgment, following your interest and passions, and staying open to new ideas and new ways of thinking. It's sometimes easier said than done but lean into new situations and concepts with the notion that it's not only interesting but could help keep you vital. We've all heard stories about someone who worked so hard to accomplish an amazing career, only to retire and then develop a debilitating illness or die early.

When we lose our sense of purpose—perhaps through judgment of what purpose really looks like and, in this case, was present and then was lost—it can feel like purpose is no longer in your life. But as you learned, your true purpose is about the intersection of what you value most, what you enjoy doing, and what you are naturally gifted at. So, spend a bit of time noting these things to lean into your growth edge. Keep your arms and eyes wide open to new opportunities that allow you to learn, grow, or try new things. The old, perfectionist version of myself couldn't have done this without judgment. But I changed, and you can too—lean more into curiosity than certainty. Have fun on the journey of growing.

Define Yourself and Express Your Gifts

And finally, a great way to move toward your "Happily ever after" is to define yourself and express your gifts. Beyond the purpose that you previously identified in the workbook, you can choose to be your favorite self. You can lose the striving to be your "best" or "highest" Self, and choose, because it's what feels good and right to you, to be your favorite self every day.

The cool thing about being your favorite self is that you get to go with the flow, and the new things you're learning start to define this version of you day after day. Just as most cells in your body fully turn over (aka die off and are reborn), you too can be a whole new you, every week—hell, every day if you like. Over one million cells in your body die every second, and they are renewed and replaced. You are constantly changing anyway, so why not show up today as your favorite self?

And remember to live out your purpose, even if it's in the smallest of ways. It can be as simple as smiling at a stranger, calling a friend, or going for a five-minute walk in nature. Your being here and living into your joy is a great way to live on purpose—no matter how big or small. When you express yourself and your gifts, you are in an aligned state, closer to your spiritual Self. This can be an energizing, rewarding, and enjoyable practice—so go have fun being you.

What you may have noticed is that many of the keys to happiness have to do with letting go of the judgment we carry—judgment of our moods, judgment of how happy or unhappy we are, judgment of how balanced we can be versus what we should be doing.

So, there is an inverse relationship between judgment and happiness; the more we judge, the less happy we are. Speaker and author Lynn A. Robinson famously said, "Would you rather be right, or would you rather be happy?" I know what I choose. What about you? We will explore this further in the next chapter.

Recognition of your default tendency, creating more of your desired feelings now, and practicing these five keys to happiness, allows you to recognize that happiness is a choice you get to make – always. It's no longer dependent on others, on a different circumstance, or a new life. You get to be happy in your life now.

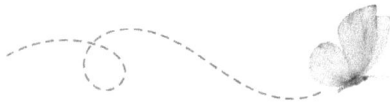

PART FIVE

THE
RETURN

Chapter Fourteen

The Rising

The Rising becomes more than what you do every day with the rising of the sun. It takes on a new meaning, to define the second chapter of life, where *you* rise. You rise from the past, which is no longer here, and no longer defines you. You rise into the wholeness and completeness of the woman that you are. You rise into the woman that you saw in the highest vision of Yourself.

Rising isn't something that just happens at the end of life, based on your beliefs, like a rising to Heaven, or everlasting life. You get to create this sense of Heaven on Earth, a sense of completeness, perfection, and serenity each and every day.

Dr. Courtney Hunt, a world leader in the field of quantum biology, mitochondrial health, nutrigenetic medicine, and hormonal health, identifies the power and the rising of the sun as symbolism in our lives for a whole new day—a whole new opportunity, a whole new perspective for which we get to face the day. And so I invite you now to let go of anything in your past that no longer serves you.

You might wonder how to do that. It's easier than you think—only a simple decision you get to make right now, today, to let it go. This doesn't mean that it will no longer resurface, but it does mean that the tug-of-war game you've been playing with this thought that no longer serves you can be surrendered. If your past is a rope, you can let go, no longer bound to the pull or push. Just let it go, trust and, maybe with a prayer, ask that it no longer consume your energy. You can receive the help you need to not pick up the rope of your past again.

RISE FOR YOU

With the rising of today's sun and the rising of the second chapter of you in your own life, choose to move into your highest, most favorite vision of You. Don't wait for the end of your life, or the start of another year, for this to happen. Make a conscious choice today.

Inevitably, because we are human, we will make mistakes. We will stumble and fall. There will be setbacks. Will you perceive them as stumbling blocks, unscalable walls, and impenetrable obstacles to your progress? Or, are they simply stepping stones, simply part of the journey of you rising into all you can be?

Biologically, we know that every day between fifty and seventy billion cells die off to become renewed into an ever-changing version of ourselves. Every seven years, we are almost completely renewed by regenerating cells having died and turned over. So, this isn't just something to envision and hope for. This is a reality of a new you today, newer than you were even last week. With your daily rising, you get back up, you keep going, you keep on the journey.

Make a point to check in on yourself to make sure you aren't falling into old habits of blindly following something or someone else's expectation of you, or anything that feels less than good to you. You deserve to feel good, confident, and great in your own skin and body in this lifetime.

When you check in with yourself—day to day, moment to moment—you can stay close to this aligned, rising, spiritual part of You.

RISE LIKE A FLOWER

The life of a flower starts as a seed, buried deeply, hidden from existence. It moves its way through the crud, dirt, worms, and soil to turn into a lanky stalk, then eventually it reaches its full, beautiful potential. That potential is the flower, its greatest beauty for us all to see, appreciate, and relish. It's delicate, radiant, vulnerable, and gorgeous in its fullness.

Yet, inevitably, it will start to wither. It will wilt and shrivel, moving back into itself, back to the ground, to the earth, to rest awhile before it starts the whole process over again the following season.

I'm pretty sure the flower as a seed isn't frustrated that it feels invisible to others, stuck in mud and "shit," waiting for the future when it can be seen and appreciated. I'm certain the lanky stalk isn't wishing it were older and more beautiful. The fully-bloomed flower isn't worried about how long it will stay pretty, how to preserve its petals, or wishing for the "good old days" when it was tall and lanky. It's not worried about what lies ahead, how it will change and transform. The wilting flower isn't stuck and reliving the past of what once was, now bitter that it's not as full, colorful, and vibrant as it once was. The flower just is.

What I challenge you to do is to view your life as the life of a flower. As opposed to viewing it as one time where you bloom, and experience your radiance, followed by a slow decline toward death. What if that cycle is more frequent than we give it credit for? What if the life of a flower is not a symbol just for our life of growing, blooming, and dying, but about multiple iterations of this journey?

Your life and body die multiple times over, as cells are renewed and replaced.

What if we view the lifespan of a flower through a twenty-four-hour lens? What if your day today, or your morning tomorrow, is a full journey of rising from the seedling that sprouts out of bed, awkward at first, to then enjoy whatever beauty is in your day? As the day comes to an end, you start to wind down, relax, and grow tired before you return to the seed of your bed to rest and then start the whole process anew, tomorrow.

When you remember the life of a flower, you can choose the symbolism that best supports you in your journey. The biggest piece is presence. The flower just is. It's not reminiscing about days gone by, or longing for the future. It's without judgment.

Any time you see a flower going through its season and cycle—on a walk, in nature, or in your home—it can serve as a reminder to you of your daily rising. It is your sign that your ability to be present, and your own rebirth of awakening to new levels of consciousness, looks different from season to season. It's all part of the natural contraction and expansion of our universal energy source. And this is how rising occurs day after day, year after year, lifetime after lifetime.

LOVE OVER FEAR

In addition to your pursuit of feeling good, notice whether you are making choices in your life that are rooted in love or fear. This has been an integral piece of decision-making in my life that I'd love to share with you now, and it's really quite simple. When you are choosing out of love, it's calm, connected, clear, creative, and confident. It might feel courageous and compassionate, or spark your curiosity. These are the "8 C's of Self" as identified by Dr. Richard Schwartz as part of Internal Family Systems (IFS) therapy, and are key qualities that represent a healthy Self.

All these things can only come from the loving, higher Self of God, Universe, Source within you, whereas when you're choosing out of fear, you are out of alignment. There is something in society, or someone's expectation, that is making you think you need to do, or be, something different in order to be okay. Yet, that was never the Truth of who you were. You were already born perfect, whole, and complete in who you are.

You know if you are choosing out of love or fear, based on how you feel. When you feel good, it's love. When you feel bad, it's fear. That's your first indicator. For me, fear-based choices feel like "I shoulds," and create anxiety and tension in my shoulders. Take a moment to consider how you feel physically when you are making choices based on fear, versus a calm, confident inner knowing.

This idea of rising, creating inner radiance and beauty within you is about checking in daily with how you are feeling. It's no longer about others' focus, and doing things for the sake of them feeling better. This is about how YOU feel.

One of the ways I support my inner radiance with the rising of the sun each day is to set my intention and note what I appreciate in my life, as soon as I wake up. If you didn't do this previously, I invite you to download this gratitude practice to use for setting your intention and direction for your day.

kindlcoaching.com/
aob-resource

Our final thing—and this is a big topic—is around forgiveness. Let's dive into that next.

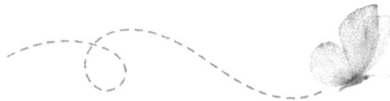

Chapter Fifteen

Integrate and Accept

As part of your daily rise into the woman you are becoming, you do not need to leave your past fully behind. You have let go of the challenges that no longer serve you today, yet can be grateful for much of your journey. There is no need to discard the woman who brought you so much joy, love, opportunity, and experience in your life. She is a warrior. She has served you well. She got you to where you are today, and she is beautiful.

So, instead of discarding or disregarding her, you get to integrate all the joy and wonder she brought you, and forgive her for her shortcomings. She was doing the best she could with the information and resources she had at the time. It is only in hindsight that you can view any prior action she took as a "mistake," by comparing the outcome to what you had hoped for. Instead of judging for mistakes made, and being consumed by them, what if you decided to accept her in a way that allows you to learn, grow, and become even stronger as the rising woman you are.

What if instead of judging her, you love and appreciate her for all she has been courageous enough to brave, committed enough to endure, and strong enough to survive? What if you could forgive her, fully, completely?

FORGIVE FOR YOUR FUTURE

One of the most powerful ways to integrate and accept not only past experiences but also your life, in general, is to forgive. We are all doing the very best we can. You and I are both doing the best we know how to do.

There are no mistakes.

And yet, if we are observing someone who is not living up to the standard we learned, it can be easy to judge. We can look at them and think, "Of course they can do better. They should know better. What they are doing is not okay. It's wrong." We are back in judgment. Our energy moves back to catabolic energy. In this low-energy place, we don't feel good.

We might feel subconsciously guilty, or more anxious, for having judged. The quick "high" of a righteous judgment of another only hurts us in the end.

As part of the rising, integration, and acceptance of yourself to feel more beautiful, you must learn to forgive. Learn how to forgive yourself. Learn how to forgive others. Learn how to forgive past experiences with the recognition that not only are we all doing the best we can, but also that when we know better, we do better.

Again, there are no mistakes.

Take a moment to think back to a time in your life when you regret something. If you really remember and consider who you were in that moment, with all of life's stressors at the time, it's almost certain that, in that moment, you were doing the very best you knew how to do. You made the best decision you could with the information you had. It's only in hindsight that you get to see that the outcome wasn't as favorable as it could have been; this hindsight is where your judgment comes from.

What if you took a moment to acknowledge what you learned from that difficult experience, and how you are a different, stronger, and better woman today as a result? If you live trusting that there are no mistakes, only opportunities to learn, grow, and rise, then it's easier to forgive in knowing we are all just doing the very best we can with the information that's in front of us.

Forgiveness can be the one thing that changes everything.

The natural evolution in life is a beautiful thing. Our parents did the best they knew how, given the way they were raised and what they had available to them. They made incremental changes to do better with us then the way they were raised. As we learn and grow, we too can take the good, the lessons learned, and bring them forward. Although we are inevitably making missteps along the way, we are doing our best. It is certain our kids will have their own learning and growth, evolving to stretch beyond even what we are able to learn. So, why not forgive those you love and yourself as part of this natural evolution?

In order to do this, review the Chapter 11 workbook exercises with Michael Singer and Gabrielle Bernstein, to integrate and accept what has happened in your life, even if it's painful. This practice of acceptance instead of resistance is a powerful way to move on from the things that you have not yet forgiven. This practice will lessen the grip your prior experience has on you, that is keeping you stuck from your rising.

Remember to check in with yourself to get back to a place of acceptance when things get judgmental or tough. If you feel good, keep going. If you're feeling bad, adjust course, or do whatever supportive internal work feels right to get you back to your good feeling, even if it's a minute change. By noticing and tuning into how you feel, you can establish a trusting, reliable barometer for your life.

THE UNHAPPY JUDGE

The less you judge, the happier and more present you will be. The more you judge, the more unhappy and anxious you will be. It's counterintuitive but important to remember.

Everything we judge in someone else has truth in our lives. Others are mirrors for a repressed part of us we're unwilling to express or admit to because we're afraid. When I envy or judge a woman who has more money than me, or seems more successful or beautiful, I'm not recognizing the beauty or success in my own life. I'm "othering" myself.

I'm operating out of lack, feeling different and less than. I am not standing in the truth of who I am. Similarly, when I judge my former boss for the way she acted or how much she hurt me, there's a truth that I, too, have done hurtful things and acted inappropriately.

Instead of judging others, which ultimately makes you feel more isolated and alone, I invite you to notice when you are judging. Then, look inward to recognize that part of yourself you are judging in another. Instead of saying, "Oh, I could never do that," think of a time where you stood up for yourself by stepping into your power. The truth is that we are not as alone, as unique, or as separate as we think. The more we can find the common threads that bond us, and the resultant compassion for

143

others, the freer we feel because we see our humanity in others. We see it in ourselves. We become inherently more forgiving, and happier in the process.

I have sometimes judged my daughter for how much she eats, and yet there's a part of me that has always felt afraid of being overweight, that I should control the amount of food I eat. So, I could stay stuck in this pattern of blaming her for not listening to her body, or recognize that I, too, don't fully trust or listen to my own body. I have been living with some fear that if I do not eat healthily enough, exercise regularly, or maintain my outward image, that I am somehow not enough. I have been carrying my same limiting beliefs and limited thoughts, and projecting them onto my daughter. In this recognition, I see a freeing beauty in who she is, as a young girl who knows and trusts herself and her body. She even giggles at her belly, squeezing it in pure joy and laughter. She's so funny about it. She could probably do stand-up comedy and draw laughter from a crowd when she rubs her belly against a window and calls it her "mating dance."

She's so full of life and loving acceptance of her body. If anything, I can learn from what she is teaching me instead of giving her a reason to doubt herself due to what I've imposed as right or wrong, good or bad. So, my commitment to myself and my daughter is that I will use this experience as a training ground to learn that I have been judging unnecessarily. Instead of judging her,

I will see myself in her. I also overeat when I'm stressed, and that's okay. When I can trust my body, and she can trust hers, we will always be brought back to equilibrium instead of feeling "less than".

As we complete this section, head over to the workbook to recall judgments you have made of others, to then see yourself in the judgment. This can be a difficult exercise, yet a critical first step in releasing the judge in you for the sake of greater happiness and self-acceptance.

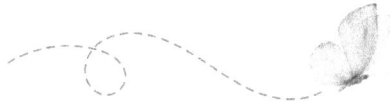

Chapter Sixteen

Full Circle

While writing this book, my family had the incredible opportunity to go on an African safari—this trip changed me. We spent most of the summer preparing—from vaccination, to packing appropriate safari colors, to reading about the wild animals and how to interact safely. I might have prepared logistically but was nowhere near prepared for the life-changing experiences we had.

Being in the wild, in the middle of the Serengeti, with zebras outside our tent, and the sound of lions nearby at night, was the most immersed in nature I've ever been. We were fully dependent on our guides for our safety, and on the Masai warrior who escorted us to and from our tent after dark with nothing but a flashlight and a poisonous arrow for his bow, in case he should have to ward off a hungry lion or startled cape buffalo.

In Arusha, Tanzania, we were given the opportunity to visit a public school. When we got out of our guided vehicles, covered in dust from the dirt road, we were met with the bright smiles of the headmaster and a few students. These young students all wore school uniforms; some were tattered and ripped, all were dusty and worn.

Many of the kids walked several kilometers to get to and from the school, bringing their cup with them so they could have a scoop of porridge for their daily lunch. Everyone had to pitch in to help clean the room before they left for the day, and gather wood for the next-day's fire to cook their daily porridge. They had so little, yet showed so much joy in their smiles, hope in their eyes, and love to give to their privilege of learning. These children taught me so much. We were overcome with joy and laughter in visiting with them, even though they knew little English, and we knew little Swahili. Our guides helped translate for us, but the truly rich communication came from the shared smiles, high fives, and fist bumps, and the palpable joy being in their presence. They were such beautiful children, inside and out. Their joy, laughter, and beauty radiated outward for all of us to see, feel, and experience.

I learned from these children, and the people of Tanzania, that as long as basic needs are met, joy and happiness—the things that really matter—can still be chosen. Even if you have to walk several kilometers to access water, wash your school clothes in a muddy stream, or forage for your next meal. Their external experience looks difficult, and should they fully depend on that alone for happiness, they would be unhappy, perhaps depressed, by the rigors of daily life.

Yet the people of Tanzania we encountered were grounded in family, community, and purpose. They choose love. They chose joy. They live with nature daily. Their culture is rich, yet without all the excess that we often consider prerequisites for a "rich" life. The people of Africa taught me that when all the excess of material things and a busy schedule are stripped away, what really matters remains—a rich culture, authentic people, and an openness to sharing love. The love shared from and with the kids on that school visit to Arusha will stay with me forever.

At the end of our two weeks in Africa, it was time to say goodbye, for now, to this rich culture and these beautiful people, to the life-changing lessons amid the wild and untamed nature of the Serengeti. We were dreading saying goodbye to our guides, as they had begun to feel like family. When it was time, our guides showed us how love can be shared and given freely—without attachment—through hugging our children and telling them they loved them. They loved us, because they choose love over differences, judgment, and fear. And we loved them. Through hugs and tears that lasted upwards of forty minutes into our airport goodbyes, we felt the richness, the beauty in our hearts that had been gifted from the people we'd met. Our hearts were full, and forever changed.

So, as we prepare to say goodbye for now, please know that you have what you need to move forward: self-love. Love is everything. To fully get there, you may need healing or self-forgiveness, but when you lean into love, you will live a rich and beautiful life.

So often, we withhold love as though it's a finite resource. But the truth is, there is plenty of love to give. You give it to your parents, spouse, kids, friends, and extended family. It is now time to give it to yourself as part of coming full circle. Love is not a limited resource. The more love you give, the more you receive. So, why not give more to yourself, as you freely give to others? Give love to everybody. When you stop operating from a place of scarcity and the belief that as you age, you will become less than, you will be reminded, instead, about the truth that you have everything you need within you.

So, you can choose to focus on lack, or to focus on the beauty within each day, the beauty within you. With the rising of the sun, notice the blessings in your life, the physical, mental, and emotional things about yourself that you truly appreciate, including your beauty. It's time to stand in that, to love your beauty, both externally and internally.

If you find it inauthentic, or too much, to just "love yourself," I imagine there is still some self-forgiveness that needs to take place. That's okay. It's a journey.

Yet remember that judging yourself less, so you can fully embrace your Age of Beauty today and everyday, is a crucial part of learning to love yourself on this journey. Remember that you are being guided, not judged.

As we wrap up *Age of Beauty*, I want to recognize and celebrate you for the steps you have taken to feel truly and authentically beautiful in your own skin and in your own life, regardless of age or external circumstance. Like all things, change is gradual and takes time, and true change requires work. Yet it is the journey through the change, while challenging at times, that makes it all worth it. You are worth it.

You've embarked on this journey and committed to yourself for meaningful change. This is something that must be celebrated. Congratulations on all the growth and progress you have made through your commitment to yourself, and through the recognition that *you* matter. You deserve to feel beautiful, each and every day, inside and out. When you forget much of what you have learned in this book and workbook, as I know you will—because you're human—I invite you to come back to the section that best supports you to reflect upon what you learned and get you back to baseline.

As we come full circle, it's important to remember that you were born perfect. You are perfect. There is nothing within you, or about you, that needs to change. Any expectation of another, or pressure from society, or defining role, or judgment that has been cast to define you or, perhaps, send the message that you are not enough, simply is not true. When you change the narrative in your mind and, instead, see the perfection in your own beauty, each and every day, you remind yourself that you truly have everything you need to have a life you love, right here and right now.

That said, if there is part of you that knows you need to take this one step further to fully ingrain the belief that you are truly beautiful, and ready to fully own and love that about yourself, head to kindlcoaching.com to learn about my current programs. Connect with me there to discuss potential opportunities to work together 1:1, perhaps in a group format, or whatever best suits you.

Again, thank you for committing yourself to this book, to this process and to your own Age of Beauty.

I look forward to seeing you in your light.

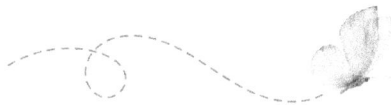

RESOURCES

Bernstein, Gabrielle. *The Universe Has Your Back: Transform Fear to Faith*. Carlsbad, CA: Hay House, 2016

Brown, Brené. *Daring Greatly: How the Courage to Be Vulnerable Transforms the Way We Live, Love, Parent, and Lead*. New York: Gotham Books, 2012

Brown, Brené. *The Gifts of Imperfection: Let Go of Who You Think You're Supposed to Be and Embrace Who You Are*. Center City, MN: Hazelden Publishing, 2010

Dyer, Wayne. *The Shift*. Directed by Wayne Dyer. 2009. Hay House Films.

Hartmann, Stacy. *Metaconscious Entrepreneur: How to Harness the Unlimited Power of Consciousness and Energy to Grow a Wildly Successful Business That Changes the World*. Bloomington, IN: Balboa Press, 2021

Singer, Michael A. *The Untethered Soul: The Journey Beyond Yourself*. Oakland, CA: New Harbinger Publications, 2013

Waldinger, Robert, and Harvard Medical School. *The Harvard Study on Adult Development.* Ongoing study since 1938, Harvard Medical School.

Winfrey, Oprah. "Your Life Is Whispering to You: Are You Listening?" *Oprah Daily*, July 18, 2021.

Acknowledgments

I am immensely grateful to my husband, Dustin, for supporting me on this soul-expressing journey of writing my first book. I could not have done it without your love and tolerance of me in this process. Thank you to our children, Carson and Elle, for pushing me to become the woman I am today.

Thank you to Momma Gardner, Eric Gardner, Lynn Akerberg, Lon Akerberg, Connie Greenberg, Breah Ostendorf, Stacy Marquardt, Larissa Soehn with Next Page Publishing and her amazing team, including Ruth Fae and Amy Vogel, the women in Age of Beauty book club including KT Anderson, Kristen Charette, Jennie Oko, Therese Dlugosch, Ruth Johnson and the ModernWell community, Julie Burton, Madison Hulett, Jasna Burza, Stacy Hartmann, Jason Gracia, my many prior clients who taught me what it means to age beautifully, Angela Divine, and my wonderfully supportive group of friends who offered me encouragement along the way.

Thank you.

www.ingramcontent.com/pod-product-compliance
Lightning Source LLC
Chambersburg PA
CBHW052114030426
42335CB00025B/2981